D1157394

BODY FREEDOM DAY

When a Clothed-Minded World Unraveled

by
Stuart R. Ward

Copyright © 2004 by Stuart R. Ward

All rights reserved. No part of this book shall be reproduced or transmitted in any form or by any means, electronic, mechanical, magnetic, photographic including photocopying, recording or by any information storage and retrieval system, without prior written permission of the publisher. No patent liability is assumed with respect to the use of the information contained herein. Although every precaution has been taken in the preparation of this book, the publisher and author assume no responsibility for errors or omissions. Neither is any liability assumed for damages resulting from the use of the information contained herein.

This book is a combination of fact and fiction. People, places, organizations and events dated 2003 and earlier are real, the quotes actual. Names and events dated past the year 2003 are real persons, places, and planned events fictitiously treated or purely products of the writer's imagination.

ISBN 0-7414-1945-9

Cover painting by American artist George Bellows

Published by:

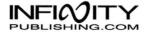
PUBLISHING.COM

1094 New Dehaven Street
West Conshohocken, PA 19428-2713
Info@buybooksontheweb.com
www.buybooksontheweb.com
Toll-free (877) BUY BOOK
Local Phone (610) 520-2500
Fax (610) 519-0261

Printed in the United States of America

Printed on Recycled Paper

Published April 2004

For C.J., who believed

And the gang at the Springs—past & present.

Acknowledgments

Greatly indebted to The Naturist Society, from whose quarterly periodical, *Nude & Natural: The Magazine of Naturist Living*, and booklet, *205 Arguments and Observations in Support of Naturism*, the majority of quotes, facts, and information on all things naturist were freely borrowed. (I take responsibility for any inaccuracies.)

Some of the bumpersticker, banner and t-shirt slogans are original; others borrowed; credit here to whoever first thought up the latter; you know who you are. The same to whoever thought up that brilliant phrase, *clothed-minded*. A tip of the hat to Arlene Donanelly for her HBO documentary film, *Naked States*, (Juntos Films, 2000) on Spencer Tunick's nationwide nude photo shoots, for brief quotes used; thanks to Ted of B2B, for the pointers and cautions.

To Candace, for her bright openness and support; to Tamy, for encouraging completing the project; to Athena for her wisdom; to John, Ron, Diandra, and Marilyn for early feedback; to Mary, for letting me help; to Cheryl, for her trust; to Dolores, for her keen enthusiasm; to Marcia, for her input; to Bruce, Peaches, and the rainbow family for setting an example; to Elizabeth and Joe, for suspecting a writer lurked in me.

Thanks to the team at Infinity Publishing for running a tight ship; to Charles Daney, both for his collection of pithy quotations, some of which head the chapters, and his *Weekly Nudesletter,* which provided valuable research material; to Steve A. Brown, who kindly checked his Georgia University archives; and to the computer technicians, who patiently helped me figure out my new laptop by phone all the way from Bombay.

◈ CONTENTS ◈

i

◈ Editor's Foreword ◈

I submit the following manuscript to a skeptical public—
make of it what you will. I'm doubtful of its authenticity
myself, yet found the contents so startling I felt compelled to
publish it. Overall, its supposed origin seems so patently
absurd, its contents so far over the top and off the wall, many
will dismiss it outright. Yet parts of it ring true and may
leave you, wondering—as it did me briefly—*what if...* And
even if it doesn't, there's enough food for thought here to
merit attention anyhow.

Let me back up a bit. I run a modest home-based book-
publishing service. Mostly self-help, biography, popular
culture—sometimes offbeat subjects no one else will
publish. I keep a Martin Luther King quote perched over my
desk: "Human salvation lies in the hands of the creatively
maladjusted." It was undoubtedly my reputation for printing,
shall we say, *unusual* volumes on occasion that led a
somewhat excited man to my door one day. He was dressed
lightly, considering the sharp autumn chill in the air. He had
a determined look in his eye, like one on a mission; I'd seen
it before. *What now?* I thought. He held up a slim blue book
with bright gold lettering and solemnly handed it to me.

"I think you may want to publish this," he said.
"Looks like I'm too late. It's already printed," I joked.
He was gracious enough to smile. "Check the title page."
I dutifully flipped open the cover. "'*Body Freedom Day,* by
Zet Quimby.' Odd title, unusual name, but...so what?"
"But check the copyright."
I did—and did a double-take. "Okay, what's the joke?"

"It's no joke. At least, not that I can figure. Want to hear the story?"

Curiosity peaked, I said sure and ushered him in my home office, offering him a seat by the fire blazing in my glass-fronted woodstove and some fresh coffee, both of which he gladly accepted. *This ought to be good,* I thought, knowing there could *be* no reasonable explanation.

The page had read 'Copyright © 2056.'

"My name's Sun," he said by way of introduction, warming his hands. "I know this'll sound nuts, but this book found *me*. Now, I hope you won't be shocked. I'm of that persuasion labeled a naturist, or nudist—whatever you want to call people who like loosing their clothes now and then." I thought, *Oh, boy, I get them all.* His sincerity and forthright manner gave me pause, though.

"I was up at a remote lake in the High Sierras a week ago for a mini-vacation—skinny-dipping and clothes-free relaxation. It was nice at first but when it clouded I decided to keep warm by hiking along the trail by the lakefront. I sensed I was the only one there so late in the season, and so wouldn't startle anyone being out of uniform, as it were. I came to another beach clearing and spotted a sign-bearing tree at the far end. Curious, I walked over. The sign, barely legible, and hand-painted, read: "Posted - No Nudity.' It was obviously home-made, the two ens reversed.

"Now, standing there naked as a jay—the very same squawking all about me—looking at this sign in the middle of nowhere telling me my lack of clothes would not be abided gave me pause. Then I remembered. Forestry used to lease lakefront lots there to vacationers to build simple cottages on for a dollar a year, until they ended the arrangement and the buildings were removed. I could picture it: Maybe ten summertime dwellers and most were okay with the occasional day-tripping skinny-dippers on their far shore, but one or two were up in arms and posted this sign, and no doubt others long since removed by rangers, taken as souvenirs or maybe used to feed campfires. Chuckling and thinking, *no problem now*, I strolled back to my spot. The sun had come out again and I sat looking over the water, reflecting on how people could get so bent out of shape over others getting shucking their clothes now and then in the great out-of-doors.

"It was funny, but also maddening. A friend of mine had just been ticketed for nude sunbathing over in Hawaii. You believe that? 'Come to Paradise' they tell you. 'Sun your Buns in Hawaii' the tourist shop bumper stickers tell you. Then they slap a fine on you when you try to. It's like *The Emperor's New Clothes* in reverse: People acting all ecstatic in their hundred dollar swimsuits splashing in the waves amid their $300-a-day vacation spots, while the child this time is pointing and yelling, "Look, Ma, they're bathin' with their *clothes* on!"

"*Anyhow*," he added, sensing my impatience to cut to the chase, but obviously not to be rushed, "my mind was in a quandary over the absurdity of humans' seeming inability to accept their own bodies. With the sun radiating on me and the lake water gently lapping the shore, I found myself slipping into a deep meditation, envisioning how nice it'd be in a body-positive world, where clothing was always optional. Time seemed to stop. I don't know how long I was gone, but I was brought back suddenly by a poof sound at my feet."

"Don't tell me. The book."

"The book." He looked chagrined over my quick deduction and obvious disbelief. "I suppose I can't blame you for not believing me. I wouldn't have believed it either, if it hadn't happened to me. But it did, and I tell you this book—

v

absolutely *not* there a second before—suddenly rested on the ground in front of me.

"And how many joints did you say you'd smoked?" I know, it was mean.

He ignored the dig as if not even hearing it. "The thing just manifested," he said in wonder as he starred at the dancing golden flames through the stove door's glass. "Unbelievable as that sounds, *it simply manifested.*" He turned and fixed me with a gaze of such intense earnestness I had no doubt *he* believed that was exactly what happened. "Listen," he said, "Just read the book through. Tell me what you think. I'll make it interesting. I bet you a dinner—winner's pick—you'll want to *re*-print it."

I was always up for a new read, especially with a friendly wager attached to it, although this one seemed more out there than even I was used to. I said I would and he left, to return in a few days. I finished up some work I was doing when he came—proofing a manuscript called *Downwardly Mobile in Style and Grace*—and picked up the book again. Funny. I hadn't noticed before, but the binding material was a kind I'd never seen. And the pages—they had an unfamiliar feel to them. The text font was one I wasn't familiar with either. Peculiar.

I settled into my favorite chair by the fire, fresh mug of coffee in hand, and began reading. The introduction stopped me cold—there was that 2056 date again. *Preposterous,* I thought. Then, in marked contrast, the first few chapters seemed entirely plausible: A brief speculation of the advent of clothes and twentieth century wear; a thumbnail history of nudism and naturism in the United States; and recent nonsexual nude trends and events—all of it apparently verifiable fact, I discovered, after doing some fast checking.

Then dates began to spill into our future; the writer would have us believe our *future* was his *past*. And the social events recounted…No. I'm sorry. It was too fantastic. Future time aside, who would believe there could ever be a nude streak by a multitude through a major city? Or a quantum leap in body attitude and semi-acceptance of public nudity? Right. The work, obviously, was the product of someone's overactive imagination. I tossed the book aside, thinking generously it might have publishing value as fantasy at least.

The next day I absently thumbed the binding material and started wondering. If only to satisfy my curiosity, I called over a scientist friend to microscopically analyze a sample tiny cut for me. He couldn't determine the material, saying it was a molecular compound he'd never seen before. Same with the paper. Unsettling. While I actually found a Zet Quimby listed in the phone book, and on calling him and explaining the reason, he was duly intrigued, he denied having written anything. Later, checking out the publisher, Peace Planet Press, I found no such publisher listed. Their supposed location, Ocean City, Idaho, I couldn't find anywhere in the atlas. *Ocean City, Idaho*?

Despite myself, a part of me began to wonder. This seemed too much effort for an anonymous prank. What if humanity, sometime in the future, actually discovered the technology for teleporting inanimate objects back through time? What if this book indeed *was* a voice from the Future? A cultural record sent back to us into the hands of Sun for some unknown reason? A wild thought I couldn't entirely dismiss, though God knows I tried. I read parts of it again and found I was gaining little insights on a subject I'd really never given much thought to before; nudity is such a private, delicate subject, one so often inextricably tied to sex—as the book pointed out—that it was indeed seldom the topic of dispassionate, rational conversations. Maybe it had more than fantasy value, after all.

When Sun returned I told him of my research efforts and the outcome; if he was surprised he didn't show it. I admitted I was indeed enough impressed with the book to want to print it—or re-print it, to believe his story. But only on the condition I add this explanation and disclaimer. And, of course, make thorough efforts to determine no one actually had a bona fide copyright on it and protect myself accordingly should someone ever come forward. Though he was frustrated I couldn't bring myself to believe his story despite the supporting evidence, this basically satisfied him—as did the meal I'd spring for later; he'd choose Italian.

In talking over the book's contents with Sun, I came out and sheepishly admitted I was one of the "closet nudists" the book talked about. I said reading it started giving me a new perspective on nakedness. We talked a long while then, by the wood stove. Sun made his own eloquent case for shucking clothes more often. Duly impressed, I asked him if he might write down some of his thoughts, tying them to the drift of the book, for this preface. He did. A week later he brought in the following, which I'm happy to include here in full:

Who hasn't wondered what it would be like if we could go naked in everyday life? Some believe that in our heart of hearts we are *all* natural-born nudists. That, were the world a gentler place—*far* gentler, filled with positive body acceptance for ourselves and each other—legions of current "closet nudists," not to mention untold millions of practicing nudists, would walk about with few or no clothes in warm weather and think nothing of it, except how natural it felt.

Strict social convention, however, taught us at early age we *must* wear clothes, that it's uncivilized and indecent—even unnatural—not to. It drums any nudist inclination out of us, or tries to. But many maintain that, as the human species is part of nature, and nakedness the natural state, a frustrated nudist lurks in us all. For some, it's just below the surface; for others it's buried deep. Alas, we have become so far removed from feeling one with nature that many blanch at the thought of being naked with others besides lovers, unless indulging in a fantasy. It simply isn't done.

While many absently dismiss our mandatory-compulsive clothes-wearing as the price we pay for being "civilized," others see this condition as a four-hundred pound gorilla in the room clothed-minded persons will not even acknowledge—even though, to dedicated naturists, it may as well be dressed in an electric-chartreuse jumpsuit emblazoned with a Clothes R Us logo, six-inch heels, sporting a purple wig, Raiders cap and Elton John sunglasses.

It would be simplistic to deny that nudity and sex often go together—this of course being the conventional reasoning back of banning public nudity. It would be equally simplistic, though, to treat them as synonymous, *as many do.*

Granted, it's a thin line between sensuous and sensual. Is one indulging in sexual behavior by relishing the physical pleasure of a bath or shower? Most everyone would say no. But what about skinny-dipping to enjoy the water without a swimsuit? Or nude sunbathing to enjoy the sun's radiance all over?

Some insist even these innocent and therapeutic pleasures constitute indecent behavior, if seen by others. But what really gets body-phobics' undies in a bunch is *socializing* these activities, getting together with kindred spirits, refusing to cave to entrenched body shame. They assume Rabelaisian sex orgies in the making. Cut off from their fuller physical selves, they cannot fathom the positive body acceptance socialized nudity fosters—or just don't care, since it upsets the status quo.

It strikes naturists as purely wrong not being allowed to get mindfully naked more often without consequence. It's a denial of one of life's most basic freedoms—*the freedom to be our natural selves*, stripped free of cloth—man-made materials which, on every warm day, serve only to reflect a wrong-headed, perverse judgment against the integrity and decency of our own biologic beings.

The good news: This irrational attitude and the threadbare ruses appear to be unraveling. Growth-oriented people are fine-tuning themselves, and healing their relationship to earth, themselves and each other. A groundswell of more enlightened thinking towards nudity (and sex) in our post-industrial greening of America is gradually transforming mainstream consciousness.

More and more people believe it is only an arbitrary obedience to the Great God Conformity and lukewarm allegiance to an increasingly outdated moral mindset that keep us from freely shedding our wraps more often without guilt or self-consciousness. The automatic linking of nudity to sex by a fading social order is slowly but surely approaching a meltdown. And naturists everywhere say *none to soon*, believing mandatory and compulsive clothes-wearing is purely irrational, patently absurd, and profoundly oppressive.

To some, the freedom to be naked if you want may seem a frivolous issue to explore in any depth during our perilous times. But these are *rarified* times as well, a time when all things are coming to light. Legions of naturists, throughout America and around the world, believe it a subject fully deserving of attention.

*****

Sun shook my hand gratefully on parting, feeling he had brought the book to the right place, despite my skepticism on the book's futuristic origin. I thanked him for helping educate me on an overlooked subject and adding his generous two cents' worth. I promised to contact him when the book was ready, as he wanted to help distribute copies. He didn't want a cent for his part in it, however. In lieu, I had treated him to another dinner—Chinese—and insisted on setting it up so a portion of any book profits would go to his favorite naturist cause.

As said, the book as a whole is intriguing enough that it doesn't matter if one treats the latter part as fictional. Bear in mind, though, the material before 2004 is, indeed, verifiably *factual*. Whoever wrote it and when, whether recently—or, if you choose to believe, in the future—the person often had a laser beam on the subject.

It really made me wonder about our current body attitudes and what I've come to realize is a possible over-attachment to clothes. The book, regardless of origin, makes for an interesting hour or two's reading. And I suspect it may change the way one thinks about clothes—and the lack thereof.

Cy Green,
Editor-Publisher,
Jumpin' Junipers Press

Editor's Notes:

The reader will notice phonetic spelling on certain words, such as *tho* and *altho and enuf,* for *though* and *although and enough.* To believe the book's supposed origin, this is the accepted spelling in the future, reflecting humanity having become more rational in its English spelling at least; I let the spellings stand. Also, certain compound words which we hyphenate or keep separate, such as *bodyfreedom* and *clothesfree,* had by then apparently fused into single words.

About these fused words: The writer never defines them, so Sun offered to try defining them: *"Bodyfreedom* (and, to a related degree, *freebody* and *clothesfree)*: 'The right, freedom, and inclination to be mindfully naked as often as weather, whim, and circumstance allow, without shame; contesting as unfair, unreasonable, and oppressive any penalty or censorship from others for doing so.'

Sun also thought a few words due about the writer's use of the words *nudism, naturism, nudist* and *naturist*: "While these are all handy labels, to a degree, and necessary, they can over-emphasize the importance of going without clothes, as if it were the main event—cult practice even—rather than a small, though vital facet of one's chosen lifestyle. It's like the grandiose word *automobilist,* given to drivers when cars first became the rage, vs. the far-less attention-pinning word *driver.* Though in the writer's time this would be understood, it needs saying in ours."

Last note: If, on the remote chance the actual writer reads these words, please contact me. I've got some questions.

How idiotic civilization is!
Why be given a body
If you have to keep
it shut up in a case
Like a rare, rare fiddle?
—Katherine Mansfield,
English short story writer,
1888-1923

The line it is drawn,
The curse it is cast.
—Bob Dylan
The Times, They Are A-Changin'

There's a place in the sun,
Where there's room for everyone.
—traditional song lyric

◄ Introduction By Author ►

2056 A.D.
Mount Shasta Isle

T here was a time the tyranny of clothes ruled the world.
Clothes weren't bad, of course. Clothes were clothes. It was people in authority—*insisting* we wear them, whether or not we needed to, or wanted to. *They* could be tyrannical.

Imagine a delightful summer day: White sandy beach, bright blue ocean, gentle sunshine. The air charged with sweet sensuality. Every fiber of your being dictates shucking clothes, becoming one with the sun-warmed earth, letting the elements work their magic.

Now imagine not being allowed to.

I know some of you will refuse to believe it, but there was a time you couldn't even *swim* naked—unless you were in total privacy, isolated from anyone who might be offended by the sight of your unclad body, who would think the only *possible* reason you'd want to be naked where others might see you is to make a shameless exhibit of yourself. Even with reasonable privacy, you likely couldn't fully enjoy the nude swimming for fear of suddenly being caught at your crime.

Life was a masquerade; costumes were compulsory.

Textile laws were enforced everywhere—except at a few,

widely-scattered freebody beaches, mineral springs and resorts, and even they could feel the heat. Otherwise nice people suppressed the right of people to enjoy the day unwrapped beyond the privacy of their home, no matter how fine the weather, no matter how pleasant the surroundings, how innocent the intent.

"Nude" was a four-letter word: It rhymed with crude, it rhymed with lewd—it rhymed with rude, dude; 'twas to be eschewed, forever booed and misconstrued. No matter your mood, your attitude, or size of brood, you'd beware the prude who wanted you zoo-ed for going nude.

Anyone daring to go bare in public could face draconian consequences. People so inclined settled for disrobing only in secluded places like deserted beaches and mineral springs, if fortunate enuf to have one nearby, and, if not, only within their homes and maybe on rooftops and furtively in their yards under cover of nite when neighbors couldn't see and report them.

Others, less attuned to the simple pleasures of communing directly with nature, disregarded the wisdom of their bodies. They seemed to accept their prisons of compulsory cloth. During hot weather they might grumble, knowing they'd be cooler without unnecessary clothing, but it was simply the way things were. Clothes were our second skin. We felt *too naked*, naked—and we didn't want to get arrested. For most, the idea of being without clothes in public went so far beyond the pale of accepted behavior it beggared belief.

It was a lamentable situation.

*****

"Why are all those people wearing so much clothes, Grandpa?"

My great-grandson Zak was pouring thru one of my antique photo books which had survived The Shift intact. Our extended family was out puttering in the family solarium, enjoying a warm fall day. The picture piquing his interest was of a group of people, circa 1900, by a lakeshore on an obviously nice, if not downright hot, day. Yet they were unaccountably covered from head to foot in reams of cloth.

"They sure look like they'd be happier without all those clothes on, don't they?" he said, more than asked.

I agreed. I tried to explain the way things were then, that people almost always kept their bodies covered up, hidden from each other and even themselves—regardless of weather or locale.

He didn't understand. "Huh? That sounds silly." He had a sudden thought, maybe hoping to explain their seemingly irrational behavior. "Were they playing hide-and-seek?"

I thought a moment. "You might say that—but they weren't having much fun. It was a serious game. People who didn't play by the rules went to jail."

"*Yipes!* That doesn't sound like fun. You sure lived in funny times, didn't you, Grandpa? Hey, Mom," he said, shifting interest. "What's for dinner?"

*****

Later, Zak's initial question still weighed on me. Why *were* they wearing all those clothes? We've lived so long now in a freebody culture it's easy for new generations to not realize we ever lived otherwise. I resolved then, in the spirit of understanding bygone eras—and perhaps to indulge my writing penchant—to commit to pen and paper my knowledge and recollections of those strange, "funny" times when, amid other absurdities, going naked was deemed a crime.

At age 106, I may forget what I was going upstairs for, or where the stairs are—sometimes, if we even *have* an upstairs—but, strange to say, I vividly recall the historic event fifty years ago that helped change the world. Yes, I was there in San Francisco that glorious spring day in 2006, the day known thereafter as Bodyfreedom Day—*the day freebody awareness made a quantum leap on the planet.*

I'm no professional writer or social historian. Others have already plumbed various phases of the subject, some brilliantly. Even so, I hope to add a fresh perspective on this, the fiftieth anniversary of the milestone happening. To my layman's understanding of relevant twentieth-century trends leading to the event—necessary to gain a deeper appreciation of the day's import—I combined media reports and anecdotal gleanings from others also there, along with my own eye-witness account of that day, plus the repercussions over the next few years. I focus on the phenomenon as it occurred in the United States. My approach is a blend of academic and informal.

Today's young adults, not alive then in that clothed-minded world, may well be amazed what a huge breakthru the happening represented, in utter disbelief how hard the struggle to gain each degree of bodyfreedom we now take for granted. The times were literally *unbareable.* Those who were there know only too well how upside down, inside out, and ass-backwards things were, and maybe don't want to be reminded of it. But then, trying to make sense of the past often allows a keener historic perspective, freeing one to marvel all the more at one's place in the time stream.

I beg the reader make allowances if I seem to approach the

subject in a scattershot way. My mind *is* a bit of an anachronism—throwback to a long-vanished era and considered something of an oddity even then. If at times I seem like an old know-it-all I don't mean to be; I suspect picking up the quill sometimes brings out the frustrated professor in me.

Zet Quimby

Ω CHAPTER ONE Ω

Are you Decent?

Body Attitudes & Dress: Prehistory - 1920s

To be naked is to be oneself.
—John Berger, *Ways of Seeing*

Why did we wear clothes so compulsively for so long? How could people act so strangely—be so self-conscious about their own physical selves as to want to hide them? And, most curious, why did it take so long for humankind to cure itself of this peculiar, obsessive behavior?

A sage once said that *the cause of anything is everything and the cause of everything is anything.*

Trying to pin down exactly why we came to be such compulsive clothes-wearers—to the point it became effectually illegal *not* to wear them in public—can be a slippery slope indeed. Undoubtedly, many factors leading to such an obsessive habit stretch past the mist of recorded time. All we can do is speculate, theorize, and point out some of the most likely contributing causes that piled up, overlapping, one on top of the other, over the ages:

- Clothes, obviously, served as protection from the elements, even as they do today. Logically, people cover up when it's cold, wet or windy—or so hot the skin needs protection—and thus maintain body comfort.

- Some theorized earliest man gradually mutated from an original hairy-ape state to avoid insects infesting his thick matt. Loosing this natural, built-in warmth, he needed to replace it, and hence clothes, in the form of fashioned plant matter and animal hides. (One might wonder about the earlier clothes being called "hides.")

- Primitive man began dressing to show tribal rank, resourcefulness, signs of distinction and wealth. In a pecking-order world, clothes were crucial for showing who was who in the zoo.

- Once realizing we were in many ways different from all other species on the planet, pride made us want to distance ourselves from the rest of creation by covering our bodies—with the skins of *their* bodies. "We are not animals!"

- For those who had lived in cold climates for thousands of years, clothes-wearing became hard-wired in their genes. These tribes, often more aggressive and warlike for dealing with a harsh climate thru constant hunting and heavy meat-eating, sometimes expanded and migrated to warmer climates. Easily overwhelming more peaceful and minimally dressed, food-gathering tribes, they soon assimilated and impressed their dress style on them. As the thickly-clothed, aggressive, hunter-warriors kept vanquishing less aggressive tribes, the default appearance of humans gradually segued from naked to clothed. (Okay, this one's a stretch, but it's something to consider.)

- Among the first clothes were animal hides and furs, and for untold ages clothes were literally "to kill for," animals being killed in the process. Is it possible that clothes-wearing was, on one level, emblematic of one's hunter-aggression, and this vibration came down thru our genes, keeping even later cloth wearers more aggressive for wearing them? (Another stretch.)

- When humans migrated from warmer climates to colder

7

ones, and when climates changed over time, clothes-wearing, formerly minimal at best, became more substantial and habitual.

There are many other likely contributing causes for clothes-wearing becoming so "fashionable":

- Clothing served to provide a mutual shield from each other's undoubtedly abysmal hygiene standards.

- Clothes were useful to slow over-impulsive and irresponsible matings.

- In some eras a naked person was seen only as a wretch so poor he couldn't afford to clothe himself. No one wanted to encourage that conclusion.

- The more we wore clothes as a matter of course, the more emerging clothing merchants and fashion traders, sensing a steady, captive market in the making, scrambled to reinforce the habit, constantly impressing on us the desirability of various body covers, thus guaranteeing themselves fabulous fortunes. Eventually styles were calculated to change from year to year, necessitating going out and buying yet *more* clothes, lest one be thought unstylish.

- In our peaceful, quiet village clusters and transparent dwellings it's always inviting and safe to forego clothes if we so choose, weather permitting. Back then, modern cities were often super-compressed with millions of people living close together. Surreal scenes of loud, toxic, decidedly daunting, un-earth-friendly energies assaulted one most everywhere. People sought refuge behind solid walls to try to keep together a semblance of balanced center—and behind solid clothes as well. Wanting to go unclad amid such unkind conditions might well have been a sign of being crazy then.

- Life truly was a crazy masquerade, filled with illusion, deception, and intolerance. Wearing a disguise of clothing gave people a better chance to muddle on thru—an incognito everyday negative forces would have to work to penetrate.

- Industrialized society had pulled us further and further away from our relationship with nature, to the point many could barely relate to it beyond superficial "scenic tours," behind glass, behind clothes, behind schedule. "The manner in which people choose to clothe themselves speaks the truth of how they perceive their ties to nature," said one signing himself as Ted. It seemed the more separated from nature we became the weirder—and more compulsively—we dressed.

- It was often a hostile world. When people battled each other, wearing different clothes helped protect the body from harm and made it easier to tell who the enemy was. In more modern times it was still hostile, tho usually on a subtler level; people, no longer needing steel or hide armor, still wore clothes as shields against indifferent or unfriendly—or *too* friendly—vibes of others.

- The kind of clothes one wore were also badges of one's station in life amid a rigid, highly materialistic, class-conscious society. Different costumes for different classes, for different professions within the same class. In a time when appearance and status took precedence over substance and heart, clothes *did* make the man.

This brings us to one of the more profound factors in the advent of mandatory dress, which I saved for last—religious and moralistic reasons:

Over time mankind struggled to become more genuinely civilized and understand the divine underpinnings of his existence, realizing there was a Creator and a mysterious rhyme and reason to life. His less sophisticated mind used two-dimensional, "either/or" thinking (in contrast to the more comprehensive "both/and") to try to understand his existence, drawing hard lines between one's "higher," spiritual self and "lower," earthly self—thus creating a chronic battle between flesh and spirit.

Today we realize the importance of harmonizing *all* parts of our being, appreciating the value of each to the other in becoming our fullest, most integrated selves. Then, it seemed most people couldn't keep a handle on the flood of sensations and lusty appetites experienced when nude and/or when seeing others nude. Religious leaders feared when people listened to their bodies they wouldn't listen to God, and maybe rightly so, as humanity was possibly going thru its evolutionary adolescence of raging hormones. So we repressed the stream of sensuous stimuli bodies are sensitive to, covering them up in animal skins and cloth—and, much later, often-dubious "miracle" laboratory concoctions— thereby hiding them and also de-sensitizing the body's capacity for feeling anywhere near so exquisitely; the extreme was hair-shirts worn by certain religious devotees to "mortify" the flesh.

Earthly desires, and, by extension, nakedness, were bad. Even bathing was frowned on; in early colonial Philadelphia, one could be jailed for bathing more than once a month. The reasoning was that to bathe one had to get naked, and, being naked, one's sexual appetite was aroused, which promptly led one to running amok. Some religious sects taught people to feel ashamed at the sight of their own bodies.

As I said, I don't know the whole story. I doubt anyone does, as the subject defies easy analysis. (For a different take, read *Addictive Dress and Other Peculiar Habits,* by Rufus T. Merriweather.) S*omewhere* along the way, due to a complex accumulation of causes over millennia, earth's more "civilized" inhabitants embraced compulsory/obsessive clothes-wearing, and oftentimes body shame as well, to one degree or another. Tho I usually wasn't much of a conspiracy theorist—someone suspecting underhanded plots behind everything—I couldn't help but wonder if the sometimes-corrupted powers of Church and State *knew* they could better control, oppress and exploit the citizenry by escalating the natural tendency of its citizens to cover themselves by making clothes mandatory.

If true, if some intentionally made others feel so ashamed of their own bodies that they must always feel the need to cover them, it surely ranks as the old world's most brilliant brainwashing ever foisted by man onto fellow man. Under the guise of pious morality, corrupt and greedy powers succeeded in no less than crimping the freedom and comfort of our own bodies, and hence, our very lives.

Most difficult for people not alive then to understand is how people could be so heartless, when there was usually enuf for everyone if they had shared. Without the cooperative spirit we've cultivated, people who could, consolidated power over others—"the little people"—and installed a corrupt system to guarantee its perpetuation. It's shocking to think people would intentionally make others feel bad about themselves in order to further their own selfish ends, but they did. All the time. And in the case of required clothing it was *all in the name of decency*; God's handiwork was judged indecent and so must be shielded from offended eyes. They told people white was black and people believed it—or wouldn't dare debate it if they wanted their family's next bread ration from the church bakery.

There are undoubtedly many other factors which rendered our natural state unseemly. Suffice it to say, whatever rational reasons humankind once had for wearing clothes soon drowned in a sea of irrational ones. What started out to make us more comfortable evolved (devolved?) into

11

becoming virtual prisons, albeit soft, for *every body*.

People, living in a confusing, strange and hostile world, had succumbed to fear, guilt and power trips, becoming uncomfortable without their security-blanket of clothing. We adapted clothing as our second skin—our psychological armor—to such a profound degree we became desensitized to our real skins and painfully self-conscious about them. And, as bare skins are crucial sensors for attuning to the environment and feeling one with it, we became strangers to the land.

$$*****$$

The start of the 1900s saw people in industrialized nations incredibly over-wrapped and uncomfortable in their skins. Swathed from head to foot, they went about seemingly in denial they even *had* bodies—or feeling mighty guilty about it, anyhow. This, tho ironically, we had a dedicated skinny-dipping President at the time—Teddy Roosevelt.

The word "leg" wasn't spoken in polite mixed company; men went beside themselves at the mere flash of women's ankles. Women were super-swathed in petticoats, corsets and girdles. Under all these were panties, an item not worn by women before the mid-1830s (until then, any form of pants was deemed too masculine). Fashion dictated wearing copious yards of thirsty cloth even when ocean dipping— women risked drowning from the sodden outfits pulling them under.

By the 1910s a stuffy Victorian era was fading. With swimming becoming popular, women took to wearing more practical tank-top swimsuits, basically the same thing men wore in the water, with upper legs covered. Skirts rose to mid-calf, yet were so tight at the knees women could barely walk in them without tripping. In 1913 the modern bra was invented: A debutante named Mary Phelps Jacobs couldn't deal with her corset showing beneath her plunging neckline and designed the first modern bra with two handkerchiefs and some ribbon. "The result was delicious," she said. "I could move more freely, a nearly naked feeling..." Future designs wouldn't be so body-friendly.

While things improved, we generally remained under sway to irrational, body-suppressive coverings and the insistence they always be worn in public. *Men* could be arrested for not wearing tops at the beach.

The good thing about a situation becoming so abysmal is that it often inspires people to remedy it. The light at the end of the tunnel came with the birth of the nudist movement.

It began in Germany in 1903 by one Richard Ungewitter, with the publication of his book, *Nakedness* (apparently never released in English translation until 2004); simultaneously, the movement started thru another German, Paul Zimmermann, who opened a clothesfree facility, (Freilichtpark, or free-light park), near Klingberg, for those open to the then-super-radical idea of spending their vacation in the nude.

The movement revived the popularity of freedom from clothes that periodically, ephemerally, bobbed to the surface throughout history for various reasons. The rallying point this time was throwing off cloth restraints in order to regain health and rejuvenate the human spirit—letting sun, air, water and earth be experienced directly. When not possible outdoors, then indoors, in gyms and pools. Advocates argued clothing restricted circulation, promoted diseases, irritated and chafed the skin and caused further body discomfort by excessive heat buildup. The world of compulsory clothes had compromised the body's ability to self-regulate and self-heal.

People giving it a try discovered that in relaxing and mindfully shedding their clothes amid pleasant surroundings they indeed felt renewed. Like snakes shedding skins. The spirit-lifting exhilaration of communing directly with nature, together, free of cloth interference, was grand therapy.

Even so, nudism faced fierce resistance until World War One, when it suddenly gained droves of enthusiastic converts across Germany and Switzerland. Citizens, impoverished by the war, sought affordable recreations; getting naked in the woods was free and enjoyable. A decade later it spread to France, England and Czechoslovakia. No doubt it was also the devastating inhumanity of the war that stirred a desire to get back to nature to heal.

The 1920s found the day's youth in the United States eager to throw off more restraints of stuffy society, adopting simpler, more body-friendly clothes. Women who first dared wearing briefer bathing suits, revealing legs entirely, were promptly arrested for indecent exposure, until laws soon changed to accommodate relaxing dress standards.

The nudist movement crossed the Atlantic by way of a recent German immigrant, Kurt Barthel, in late 1929. Ephemeral pockets of freebody cultures had previously cropped up briefly in various intentional communities around the country for a century already, but Barthel's efforts were generally acknowledged as the beginning of modern, organized nudism stateside. In delicious historic irony, it took root here the same time as the great stock market crash—people started loosing their shirts the same time they were loosing their shirts.

Resistance was even more fierce in the U.S. Ninety-nine percent of Americans had never even *heard* of the concept of nudism. Altho the first nudist camp, Barthels's Sky Farm, forty miles from New York City, earned the acceptance and respect of local police as "a damn fine crowd" by working with them from its inception, others, either in less liberal-minded regions, or not trying to work with their community, didn't fare as well. Five deputies stormed one early rural nudist camp in New York State in 1930, jumping out of the bushes with pistols drawn—bearing arms on bared arms, as it were—as if in mortal fear of the naked people. That's how violently anti-body we could be. There was a word for such people: gymnophobiacs—people who had a fear of their own nudity, and that of others.

That our bodies were more than mere instruments of physical pleasure and procreation, assimilation and elimination, that they were also the earthly temples of our souls and, as such, worthy of honor and acceptance, seemed fairly lost on our more self-alienated culture. That said, tolerance by the public on the growing popularity of nudist preserves—by 1938, there were at least eighty-one active nudist groups across the country—tenuously grew along with them. It was estimated twenty percent had problems with local authorities, raids in early years and in later years restrictive legislation—actual or proposed—designed to render various nudist clubs illegal.

In due time, after court battles and attendant publicity that won over converts and sympathizers, nudist enclaves became more tolerated. So long as they kept beyond view of the disapproving, leering, and not-sure-what-to-make-of-it public and tried to meet the community at least half way they had a good chance of being left alone. But not always. Like Old West fortresses surrounded by natives outraged over white people's land invasion, nudists insulated themselves away from a public outraged by nudists' invasion of their clothed-minded domain and often fought off war parties.

People joined nudist clubs for different, oftentimes overlapping, reasons. The vast majority joined to experience the relaxation and exhilaration and health benefits which freedom from clothes allowed. In addition, many joined:

- Out of simple curiosity.
- For freedom from conventional lifestyle.
- To gain a sense of well being and self-acceptance.
- To associate with kindred spirits not down on the body.
- To get an all-over tan.
- To indulge the senses more fully.
- To allow their children to be more free and accepting of themselves and others.
- To have a pleasant and different vacation spot.
- To enjoy sports and recreation in the buff.
- To socialize free of clothes-created status.
- To foster a morality not dependent on shame and guilt.
- To experience the more honest communication social nudity often allowed.
- To experience the aesthetic joy of seeing fellow humans in their totality, appreciating the human body as a thing of beauty.
- As a way to safely rebel from a conformist world.

Memberships were kept secret and people mingled on first name only basis. Nudity was often mandatory inside the compounds, a policy as extreme as compulsory dress outside, perhaps, but understandable when you consider: In a culture obsessed with mandatory cover-up, naked people rendered themselves extra-vulnerable and sensitive and as such could feel uneasy among those secured behind the often-desensitizing armor of clothes. In 1931 the American Sunbathing Association formed to help publicize, organize and legitimize the then-daring new lifestyle in the United States.

Meanwhile, in Germany, there was new resistance to its by-then flourishing nudism: "One of the greatest dangers for German culture and morality is the so-called naked culture movement. It takes away women's natural shame and robs men of their respect for women, so destroying the conditions for real culture."—so warned the emerging Nazi regime.

Ω CHAPTER TWO Ω

A Nude Awakening

Momentous Changes: 1920s - 1970s

The body seems to feel beauty when exposed to it as it feels
the campfire or sunshine, entering not by the eyes alone but equally
through all one's flesh like radiant heat, making a passionate
ecstatic pleasure glow not explainable.
—John Muir

Back in America, hucksters and racketeers tried cashing in on the newborn nudism trend with prurient slants in ads and publications and further gave nudism a bad name. It was difficult maintaining a sense of integrity amid such a leering, condemning culture. Nudism would be equated with lewd behavior and perversion in the public mind's eye for generations. The concept was so alien and morally frightening in America that, before a court victory in 1937, one didn't have the legal right to even *advocate* the idea; such talk was deemed risking social disorder.

Men chanced arrest in 1934 by starting to go topfree at New York public beaches. They gained the legal right by the late 1930s, something women wouldn't *begin* to gain for another sixty years or so. The reasons? Male-dominated society made the rules to favor themselves. The female body, as handmaiden and nurturer of human life, is powerful; keeping it rigorously covered slowed women from embracing this strength and causing men to loose their advantage.

Also, males had so completely sexualized women's bodies they didn't want to see their breasts unless wanting to be aroused. (And if breasts didn't meet their standards of desirability they *definitely* didn't want to see them.) Since studies suggested women could be as sexually attracted to men's bare chests as visa versa, it was, needless to say, a gross injustice women were made to cover up but not men. Those into astrology believed the United States' seemingly endless preoccupation with this female anatomy stemmed from our nation's sun sign—influencing personality—being Cancer, "ruler" of the breasts. In any event, it took little stretch of the imagination to see the later advent of a ubiquitous burger chain's neon yellow arches as giant, glorified cartoon boobies thrust skyward across the land.

American society's comfort zone when it came to the unadorned human body expanded at a glacially slow pace. While nudism was taking root to varying depths in practically every civilized country, in America the seeds of bodyfreedom found relatively rocky soil—could it be because Europe had gotten rid of all its super-strict Puritans to America at our inception? Nudism here was kept rigorously contained within walled, gated communities for decades to come.

World War Two forced changes on dress. Fabric shortages spurred government restrictions forbidding extravagant ruffles and full-cut sleeves on women's wear, as well as an order to reduce fabric in women's swimwear ten percent. A halt to production of zippers and metal fasteners inspired the wraparound skirt. War's end brought out the women's bikini swimsuit—as if celebrating peace by liberating the body a bit more. It was promptly banned in Italy, Portugal and Spain and generally banned from Hollywood films until the early 1960s.

The 1950s were considered the golden era of nudism. A major court victory for freedom of the press and the nudist movement was won in 1953 by one Illsley Boone, who for thirty years was the most dynamic, colorful, and often controversial proponent of U. S. nudism. Enjoying playing David and Goliath, in one issue of his *Sun* magazine he defiantly refused to airbrush out genitals from his nude photos—the only way the post office would handle such illustrated nudist literature. When the post office refused to touch them, Boone enthusiastically appealed. In 1953, the D.C. District Court overturned the decision. From then on, the mails carried nudist magazines depicting people as they *really* were. (Of course, such relaxing of the law prompted often-tasteless, body-objectifying porn magazines to flood the market as well.)

The 50s did see a fresh enthusiasm for going nude more often—including the low-key popularity within beatnik circles—and the word being spread more easily. But nudism basically remained bodyfreedom practiced by the few, in segregated compounds, removed from everyday living, by membership only. It was progress, but we had a long way to go before more than a tiny minority, viewed askance as eccentrics at best, found the idea of getting together, free of clothes outside the home, anything but shocking or idly arousing. And skinny-dipping on public lands, why, you could get *arrested* doing something like that!"

*****

Come the hippie movement of the mid-to-late 1960s and early 1970s and the cavalry had arrived.

Each generation has fresh notions how to live, often at odds with the proceeding one, taking for granted their achievements, often hard-won, even while enthusiastically building on them as if their own. My generation seemed to come of age at a dreary, rock-bottom, time-to-drain-the-pool point in time. There existed a lock-step mentality of conventional lifestyle, a blind obedience to an intolerant State while a war raged far away that we were forcibly drafted to fight and die in. We became part of what had to be one of the greatest generational clashes the world had ever seen. (I use the royal "we." I was a fairly timid soul, outwardly at least, but always freely basked in the reflected glory of my generation.)

The most courageous and valiant rebelled against anything and everything that interfered with our living as free universal beings on the planet. A re-emergence of ancient wisdom and mystic knowledge flooded the hearts and minds of millions. Life was embraced as a miracle worthy of celebration.

Authorities were not pleased.

As we parted company post-haste with irrational old ways, the first to go were the guilt-ridden attitudes and exploitative dehumanization of the human body. We rediscovered the child within and regained a childlike sense of innocence by getting back to nature and becoming one with the earth. Uninhibited social nudity became common in such circles, both in the seclusion of nature and even in the openness of the city. The advent of guilt-free body acceptance was extraordinarily captured in the tribal musical *Hair!* Cast members removed their clothes at the end of one soaring number and brought home the simple dignity and splendor of the unadorned human body. Maybe it helped we had another skinny-dipping president in the White House—LBJ.

In 1969, John Lennon and Yoko Ono astonished the world by posing matter-of-factly nude on their *Two Virgins* music album, front and back, among other things effectively protesting the clothes-obsessed world and its all-pervasive body shame, which they *clearly* weren't buying into.

Reflecting the momentous breakthrus in bodyfreedom, many college students, in the exuberance of youth, became obsessed with streak-ins, trying to outdo each other for sheer volume of naked participants. The University of Georgia, Athens campus was determined to beat out North Carolina and on March 5, 1974, during a magical spell of exotic weather, *1,500* nude students converged. Over-reacting police, in part deciding the campus was possibly getting *too* nude, in part reacting to a heated black student demonstration waged the same day against a visiting lecturer perceived as a racist, swooped onto campus with tear gas and gnarly attitudes to disperse the crowd. The streakers undoubtedly set a new record, tho.

We quickly learned to celebrate life free of many trappings of society. Bras were burned; women, freeing themselves of "booby traps," allowed free circulation of blood and lymph again, the constriction of which by many bras was suspected linked to heart disease and breast cancer. We went bare-foot a lot, regaining a fresh connectedness with earth. Newly adopted clothes, besides being wildly cheerful—if not luxuriantly splendiferous—were often of natural, breathable fiber and/or generously loose-fitting.

Meanwhile, the Madison Avenue world of fashion reflected this flirtation with greater body-acceptance with the mini-skirt, rising to mid-thigh. Thousands of women around the world were arrested on indecent behavior charges. And that wasn't even the later, more daring micro-miniskirts and hot pants—often little more than loin cloths—the latter of which, originating with European street walkers, became briefly fashionable for more daring "respectable" women with bodies to flaunt and/or statements to make ("it's my body; I'll wear what I want").

The hippie counterculture swelled to epic proportions, affecting the lives of millions, before seeming to run out of steam by the mid-seventies. On the superficial level it appeared it had all been a dream, that people had regained their senses and re-joined the "real" world. But the precious freedom-loving seeds had been sown far and wide and found receptive soil, soon to sprout changes within the minds of open-minded millions the world over.

Ω CHAPTER THREE Ω

"It's Like Wearing Nothing"

Pushing the Envelope: 1970s - 1990s

...clothes make the man—
into a victimized pawn of the State.
—Lee Baxandall, founder of The Naturist Society

The idea of getting naked in non-sexual ways with kindred spirits and solo, both indoors and out, was by the 1970s— and definitely, by the 1980s, 1990s and early 2000s— appealing to lots of people. Soon, nude *anything* had its enthusiasts. Swimming and sunbathing, of course. But now: nude biking, hiking, running, camping, canoeing, aerobics, dance, yoga, gardening, cooking, housework, computer work, sailing, skiing, hang-gliding, kayaking, sky diving, scuba diving, driving, surfing, kite flying, acting, rock climbing, horseback riding, golf, in-line skating, ice skating, bowling... You name it. "Anything fun can only be more fun nude" was the growing sentiment.

Especially nude swimming. Bathing "suits," as such, were a modern development of the eighteenth century—1868 is one date given—created in response to greater numbers of people of mixed genders gathering at water. Before these modesty suits—"shame suits," as some called them—swimming nude or in your "skivvies" at most was the norm, especially for men.

Many of us had always felt being un-naked in water was like taking a bath with your clothes on; we were inspired to return to time-honored ways. Formerly low-key and tranquil skinny-dipping spots were soon overrun by flocks of new enthusiasts (and attendant low-life voyeurs), as skinny-dipping fever hit America. Complaints from various disgruntled locals flooded in and suddenly these once-tranquil spots were in danger of being barred to the bare.

To the rescue: Lee Baxandall. In 1975 a popular free beach (so called for one being able to enjoy it clothesfree) in the Cape Cod National Seashore was threatened with being put under textile lock. Baxandall garnered grass roots support, organized a giant nude beach demonstration and successfully kept the beach clothing-optional—a phrase he coined, incidentally, one among many. Efforts spread to coordinating with West coast free beach activists, initiating a National Nude Beach Day, and documenting information on nude-swimming areas nationwide.

Efforts expanded further to help secure bodyfreedom rights and in 1980 Baxandall founded The Naturist Society, out of Oshkosh, Wisconsin. The first issue of its quarterly prophesized a naturist culture would *"...one day decisively break through the wraps of the decadent clothes-compulsive regime."* The Society's major credo: nurturing positive body acceptance of self and others thru non-sexual social nude gathering wherever and whenever possible and appropriate—in the process gaining an increased sensitivity and respect for each other and the land. It appeared the old hippie dream lived on after all.

Earlier organizations had worked to secure legitimacy and gain participants for the walled nudist enclaves and clothing-optional resorts; pushing the envelope for the right to be naked in select *public* places was a whole new ballgame. Skinny-dipping enthusiasts had been isolated from each other and relatively powerless to protest any high-handedness by authorities deciding to clamp down on public nudity at beaches. The Society served to pull people together and champion the right to mindfully shed clothes.

Proceeding in the spirit of compromise and accommodation with the clothed world while at the same time pressing for their rights, the membership showed there was a wide spectrum of nude enthusiasts with votes and dollars who would no longer be dismissed as a weird lunatic fringe. People were entitled to enjoy their scenic public lands *fully*, not once-removed by unnecessary, often irritating wrapping that served no earthly purpose except spare the body-phobic having a cow.

Thru nude gatherings, guidebooks, legal defense and lobbying, the Naturist Society lifted a lamp for body liberation. It inaugurated Nude Recreation Week each July. Its quarterly publication, *Nude & Natural*, bore witness to trends on a global level, and explored nudity thru history, becoming a leading voice in educating and informing on vital issues and making the world a body-friendlier place.

Emerging about the same time were the high-flying rainbow gatherings. These annual alternative-culture gatherings were started by hippies holding the vision of a year-round Peace Village, an intentional rural community of grand scale; it didn't pan out back then, but something extraordinary came of their efforts, anyhow: Beginning in 1972, people from all walks of life came together each year for weeks of full-tilt summertime celebration on remote national forest lands, far from "Babylon," and shared in a hippie-rainbow dream of trying to live together in peaceful harmony. Clothing was always optional.

Held for decades, each year in a different state, its celebrants could number over 30,000. Free food, medical care, child care, and music transformed the wilderness into an instant village, one in which people shared freely and often felt safe to go about clothesfree or in abbreviated glad rags for days—weeks—at a time. These gatherings also served to help people deal with body shame, perforce, thru public privies; doing your business, squatting amid scores of people in mutual view, while daunting at first, could be a life-changing experience as much as walking around naked.

Experimental sensory awareness workshops became highly popular. They allowed numbed-down city dwellers to re-sensitize their bodies in a supportive atmosphere, and were often guided by professional therapists. To help people tune into their bodies and also help strip away any influence clothes might have in blocking growth, at least part of many classes were done in the nude.

People from all walks of life found common ground, discovering a peace, a sense of liberation and well-being that came with mindfully going bare. People felt more socially open and honest naked. Being nude was exhilarating, therapeutic and rewarding—and our right as human beings. So, while much of mainstream society settled for getting "almost naked"—certainly getting closer all the time to a state of nakedness, tho clinging to bits of cloth in token allegiance to the clothed order—others took the plunge and discovered the simple, profound liberation in being utterly, simply, nude.

Free beaches and hot springs and resorts merrily multiplied like tropical naked isles amid textile oceans. People drove and flew hundreds, if not thousands, of miles for the opportunity to experience the simple, exquisite sense of being naked among like-minded people and amid pleasant, healing surroundings.

Some mineral-spring resorts that once required public-zone cover-up embraced changing body attitudes, compromising in hopes of accommodating both those still preferring keeping wrapped in public areas as well as those now maybe wanting to get naked and stay naked. Such places could become veritable checkerboards of clothing-optional and cover-up zones. People, perforce, became adept quick-change artists: Cool here, not cool here, cool here, not cool here... It was all very schitzy but reflected the times perfectly. Was it or wasn't it okay to be naked in public?

Part of the problem hampering a smoother acceptance of nudity stemmed from the cards being stacked, not only by church and state, but by business and media as well. Some said they were all the same; those with the gold made the rules. Business and media had vested interests in their type of wares and sales slants. Strange to say now, but they seemed to *want* to keep us uncomfortable, self-alienated and insecure about our bodies. Being wrapped up and thrown off-center seemed to enable the greatest mass sales volume to "consumer units"—as shoppers were so endearingly called. By continual body objectification, automatic linkage of nudity to sex, and excessive dress, the business system made an entire industry systematically exploiting suppressed sexuality and the perpetual longing for a sense of natural being.

Movies depicting any kind of positive non-sexual nudity were scarce in America. While notable exceptions, such as *Emerald Forest*, showed how natural and unselfconscious nakedness could be, the overwhelming majority made the hardwired connection between nudity and sex every time. Or nudity and violence. Anything but peaceful, non-sexual nudity.

The frustrated yearning for bodyfreedom was manipulated by body product makers. Their spoken message: "Buy this, buy that and you'll finally feel good about yourself and be accepted by others." The stark truth: "We're shamelessly pandering to your every raging body insecurity, your every petty body obsession, your futile longing to loose your body alienation, while actually we're re-enforcing them at every turn, while offering you illusory crumbs of salvation thru our lovely products." They were like drug dealers, trying to keep us hooked on things many of which weren't really needed or were outright bad for us—products seemingly good only for draining our pocket and re-enforcing the disconnect from our real selves.

The biggest "dealers," of course, were the multi-billion dollar textile and clothing concerns. They would make us feel it our patriotic duty to go out and buy ever more of their endless textile offerings to help stimulate the economy. And, clothes-junkies that we were, we'd gladly succumb, going out hunting for new threads to drape over ourselves tho our closets be jam-packed. No problem. We'd go thru them later and donate no longer used clothing to charity to make room for our latest trophies.

The United States may have known poverty and starvation, but the poorest of the poor almost always had access to rivers of free clothing—castoffs from a swelling sea of surplus apparel. In the 1980s I'd sometimes salvage items at my local city dump, hoping to recycle them; the thrifty New Englander in me was dumbfounded and saddened by the sight of the mountains of still-serviceable things we threw out so mindlessly.

To the point: I sometimes came across maybe a dozen fresh-tossed garbage sacks, each brimming with laundered, neatly folded clothes, some bedraggled, sure, but most perfectly good yet. I thought to take them to the local thrift shop...until I learned they *came* from the local thrift shop. These were clothes the shop had maybe tried moving in their Free Box in front of the store and couldn't. All but the most destitute seemed to have more clothes than they knew what to do with. We were *drowning* in clothes. It was an inconceivable waste of resources, both human and material, and a sorry degradation of the environment.

And they could be uncomfortable as hell. The clothing

industry worked our bodyfreedom yearning to the nth degree. Cooed the voice-over in a bra ad: *"it's like wearing nothing."* Why not wear nothing instead, I always wondered (altho I later learned some women do need the body support.) Seemingly implicit in the clothing industry's promises was the understanding that real, clothing-optional bodyfreedom was never going to happen—and why would anyone want it to, *really?* But hey, here's something even *better*, only $9.95, available in a rainbow of colors, hurry, while supplies last.

Tickling the Dragon
Naturist Trends: 1990s - 2005

The vulnerability of the nude body
is a peace sign, in and of itself.

—Toni Anne Wyner, activist naturist, once arrested on Florida beach
after wrapping herself solely in an oversized copy of the Bill of Rights

Was it any wonder it took people so long to see thru the
relentless brainwashing that kept us from realizing positive
body acceptance? Mainstream media perpetuated the
negative mind-set, trivializing and marginalizing whatever
freebody incidents and happenings made it past the usual
reporting blackout. Too often they were spun into smirking,
closing sound-bites on television, and bon mot in print and
on the Internet, under headings of "Weird," "Odd," and
"Strange." Some people began to wonder if maybe the
weirdest, oddest, strangest thing of all wasn't media's
attitude on the subject.

Tenuous breakthrus were made in the U.S.: New York, Ohio,
North Carolina and Washington D.C. made it kinda, sorta
okay for women to go responsibly topfree anywhere a man
could—if they dared weather the storm of stares and hoots,
and possibly policemen acting in ignorance of the new,
untested law. Parts of Canada allowed women to swim
topfree in public pools, sometimes. Mothers could freely
nurse their babies in public, in twenty states, anyhow. Naked
street theater was allowed in Berkeley, off and on. Select
clothing-optional beaches flourished, unless shut down amid
rallying cries of family values. We saw the advent of the
thong swimsuit and the more daring women (and even a few

men) could at last sun their buns at beaches—unless they picked the wrong beach and got arrested. It often seemed three steps forward and two steps back.

Meanwhile, Europe was light years ahead of America in accepting public nudity:

- All but two beaches of Denmark's thousands of miles of coastline were clothing-optional.
- Swedish coastlines were almost as tolerant.
- In Germany, Zurich officially accepted nudity in municipal pools in 1989, after finding there was only eighteen percent opposition.
- In Munich and Zurich, office workers on lunch could sunbathe and picnic in the buff in parks right in the middle of town.
- During a heat wave in 2002, German workers opted to work nude in the office to beat the heat and it was no big deal.
- In many German saunas people were asked to leave if they tried wearing towels, swimsuits or sandals. The sauna was deemed a pure, healing freebody zone, clothing *verboten.*
- In France, a 1995 poll found that only seven percent were shocked by the sight of naked breasts on the beach; an earlier 1982 Harris poll found that eighty-six percent of French favored nudity on public beaches.
- Beach nudity was the fashion in Romania.
- England had over two million registered nudists.

Holland, Portugal, Spain, Greece…all seemed closer to mainstream acceptance of public nudity than our land of the fee…er, free. ("Wanna be naked? Nearest place is 200 miles across the state line, I hear. Forty bucks to get in—but, hey, you wanna *see* naked, come right in. No cover, two-drink minimum.")

The desire to integrate a more personal naturalness into one's everyday lifestyle was part and parcel of the larger trend towards natural living on all levels: eating healthy, seeking natural medicine and healthcare (massage, yoga, mineral baths, saunas), dedication to preserving and restoring wild nature, keeping fit, abandoning harmful products, recycling, adopting renewable energy sources...the list was endless.

By the year 2000, a national Roper Survey, commissioned by the educational branch of The Naturist Society, revealed that fully *eighty percent* of Americans were okay with the idea of having designated free beaches. Twenty-five percent admitted they had skinny-dipped and/or nude sunbathed in mixed-gender social settings.

The clothed world running government, pressured by a religious right that turned intolerance almost into an art form, was alarmed by this dismal trend. When they weren't busy throwing clothes on venerable nude statuary, they tried enacting new oppressive laws and dredging up old ones, equating any and all public nudity with indecent exposure, disturbing the peace and obscene behavior. One state tried to bring back banning men from going topfree. In 2000, Indiana passed a law in which persons found skinny-dipping or nude sunbathing on public land, no matter how remote, could not only be arrested but made to register as sex offenders. A few other states tried to follow suit, but the bills were defeated in legislature after an ever-vigilant naturist political action committee rallied forces.

One still risked ridicule and extreme discomfort, if not job loss and arrest, whenever trying to enjoy being clothesfree beyond the confines of their home and the few designated free beaches and private lands. Those who refused to cop a guilty attitude for their nudity, calling the system on its irrational body-shame bluff, became a thorny problem for the clothed-minded. To them, the very idea of not minding if one's genitals were exposed was *incomprehensible*.

Law-makers, reflecting this body-denial, turned an infuriatingly blind eye to the constitutional protections guaranteeing an inalienable right to the pursuit of happiness; our pursuit was definitely being alienated. Too bad if it gave you peace and serenity and made you feel better as a human being. Can't allow it. Can't do it. Buncha nuts. No decent person. Why, the very *idea*, ad infinitum.

It was as if their repulsion towards others' nudity mirrored some intractable alienation they felt about their own bodies. "We become what we behold," as Marshall McLuhan noted. They became outraged by others who were, in effect, storming the battlements of their own denial, threatening to shatter their long-nurtured belief that always keeping the body covered, regardless of temperature or environment, was healthy, normal, the right and proper thing to do.

However, more and more of us regained a fine-tuned sensitivity to how we lived and where we lived, what was reasonable and rational, and what was not. Some felt it a foregone conclusion we would eventually rebel, deciding the compulsory wearing of clothes was just too weird—in warm weather especially. On such days, people living in more human-friendly regions wore less and less—if not discarding clothes outright when in relaxed natural surroundings. Whenever circumstances and derring-do allowed; it always felt right. Some even took it to the streets.

In the early 1990s, UC Berkeley student Andrew Martinez, "the Naked Guy," became popular culture legend. A gentle but determined soul, he regularly walked around campus and attended classes wearing only sandals, peace symbol and backpack—and so naturally and inoffensively no one complained for a long while. (Eventually, a female student would protest she felt sexually harassed by his nude presence.)

Low-key, calm, and natural about it, Martinez, a rhetoric major, argued the right to not wear clothes: "Clothes are totally a creation of need and of capitalistic society," he said. "I don't want to facilitate the power structure with my conformity." At a Nude-in at Sproul Plaza, twenty-five joined him in getting naked after he sang The Doors' *Break on Through To the Other Side*. He told a crowd of 400, "The shame needs to be eradicated. It would be nice if everybody, around the world, would raise up their arms and take off their clothes." A growing minority of naturists around the world undoubtedly agreed wholeheartedly.

Youth in particular had a more casual, body-positive attitudes towards nudity—with the odd exception of some baggy-bottomed teen males. During warmest weather in more free-thinking regions many opted to dress in minimal apparel that seemed to say, "keeping our bodies covered is so ridiculous, but here's a few token threads to appease any lurking rag police, ha-ha. Get over it, people!" It became trendy around 2003 to wear pants so low on the hips it looked like they were sliding off, surely a sign the end was almost in sight—of mandatory clothes, that is. Semi-transparent clothes also gained a bit of popularity in some circles.

Easy-on, easy-off sandals and flip-flops became popular, making for happier feet—feet too long imprisoned in binding shoes and sweltering socks. Going barefoot found favor again as in the sixties, people rediscovering the comforting pleasure of feeling a grounding, bare connection with mother earth. Of course, one could feel *twice* as fine naked *and* barefoot as when wearing only footwear. Something about a reflexology activation of the entire body thru the soles of the feet by receptive earth fostered a sense of super-integration of body, mind and spirit we fairly take for granted now. Back then, after a lifetime of body oppression, the feeling was utterly delicious.

Group streaking among friends and various sport aficionados happened more and more. An in-line skating group, led by one Sandy Snakenberg, delighted in making periodic nude skates in and around San Francisco. As many as forty people made quick glides thru Golden Gate park without a stitch on. "The whole point is getting a lot of like-minded souls together to go out and play," he said. A dozen nude-skated across part of the Golden Gate Bridge, waving to motorists. In Seattle, nude bicyclists became an integral part of the Freemont Arts Council's annual Summer Solstice Parade; in 2003, eighty of the participants, festively body-painted and psyched with naked camaraderie and positive body-acceptance, wheeled thru the parade, some performing prankster street theater, much to the delight of spectators, young and old alike. One skit had mock policemen chasing mock nudists dressed in flesh-tone body suits.

In Wisconsin, up to 1,000 college students regularly celebrated school's end with a nite-time mile run in the buff; other colleges held similar rites every year. Neo-pagans rallied for their right, under religious freedom, to be sky-clad (clothesfree) during their coven ceremonies on public lands. Streaking inevitably went commercial. Professional streakers, running naked at events to startle and draw attention to brand names, slogans, or events plastered on their skin, earned a fee per streak from marketing companies. If it was about corporations making money, it was just business, okay; if it was for personal freedom and comfort, no way.

One summer day in 2001, a Eugene, Oregon woman, Terri Sue Webb, chose to bicycle nude thru town, believing it her right to set her own dress code. She biked calmly and inoffensively, yet was arrested for disorderly conduct. Appearing nude at her court date, she was arrested again for contempt and required to undergo psychiatric evaluation. She then challenged the court's presumption that preferring nudity was a sign of mental disorder, and nude activists rallied to her defense. She said, "To be offended by the visual appearance of another person is prejudice, akin to racism. The right to exist, uncovered, should hold precedence over the right not to view this, for the objection is irrational."

Nude protests for various causes became more common around the world—a sure way to get press, both for their cause and also for bodyfreedom. A popular ad campaign by animal rights supporters PETA had celebrities posing nude and saying, **"I'd rather go naked**...than wear animal furs." Later, some of their proactive members ran naked in Pamplona, Spain to protest against bulls being abused during the annual bull run and slaughtered for sport in the bull ring.

In November, 2002, to protest the approaching war in Iraq, the global Baring Peace project was launched by a group of forty-five anti-war women in Marin County, California. They bared at Love Field to form a living nude peace symbol for the camera. In time, up to hundreds of naked people at once, throughout America and around the world, followed their example, laying down in natural settings—sand, grass, even snow—to form living nude peace signs and spell out anti-war and pro-peace messages. In Australia, 750 clothesfree women formed a giant heart on a hillside, along with "no war" spelled inside in lettering three bodies thick. Efforts to block one such nude protest in Florida was defeated when U.S. District Judge Donald Middlebrooks ruled that "nude overtly political speech in the form of a 'living nude peace symbol' is expressive conduct well within the ambit of the First Amendment."

In various regions citizens posed tastefully starkers for calendars to raise funds for worthy causes. Sales were brisk, and soon scores of calendars were available; a movie was even made about the wild success of one.

On August 4, 2002, 1,130 moms and their babies got together in Berkeley for an intercontinental nurse-in competition, beating out Australia, reminding everyone of the functionality of breasts and, in effect, demonstrating for the right of mothers everywhere to nurse in public. The event also underscored the fact that breast-feeding was regaining popularity.

In England, TFTBY—the Freedom to Be Yourself—was spearheaded by one Vincent Bethell, who spent six months in jail for his beliefs—naked, of course. He and supporters protested nude in public...for the right to be nude in public. "Legalize your physical identity," Bethell urged. "...you should not be persecuted or victimized for being born human, with a human body - NAKED!" Explaining further, he said: "...I just think you should have the right to walk down the street naked. I firmly believe that naked people should have equal rights with clothed people." The group forcefully stated their case on their website:

HUMANITY AT PRESENT IS ILLEGAL. YOUR HUMAN BODY IS NOT ALLOWED. IT IS SUPPRESSED BECAUSE YOU ARE ILLEGAL. STOP THE OPPRESSION AND LEGALIZE YOURSELF. IN REALITY, BEING HUMAN IS NOT A CRIME.

In summer of 2003, another daring soul, one Steve Gough, hiked the entire length of Britain, 847 miles—from southern England to northern Scotland—in the nude, ignoring what he saw as antiquated attitudes towards the naked body. "I am celebrating myself as a human being," he said. "We have been brought up and conditioned to think our body is something to be ashamed of. We are made to feel bad about ourselves and that is damaging society." He was arrested over a dozen times along the way, beat up, considered a shameless exhibitionist by some, and a hero of the times by others. He claimed he wasn't a nudist but wanted to "...enlighten the public, as well as the authorities that govern us, that the freedom to go naked in public is a basic human right."

Back in the U.S., the annual Burning Man festival on an ancient lake bed in Nevada was a week-long experimental community of 25,000 or so which playfully challenged participants to express themselves in ways far beyond what was normal in everyday life. Nudity, often with bright body paint, or wild, abbreviated clothing was often favored to help achieve this.

International nude-group photographer Spencer Tunick gained controversial renown by gathering up to 7,000 naked volunteers together in public places around the world over the years, orchestrating artistic, often surreal poses for the camera. "I want people to feel uncomfortable that they've demonized the body," he said. "These grouped masses which do not underscore sexuality become abstractions that challenge or reconfigure one's view of nudity and privacy." He was often arrested early on in New York City; he was welcomed in later years in such countries as Australia, Chile and Spain. Said one enthused first-time poser in Texas: "it was like I'm freed to be me."

Forces were polarizing. At the same time historic breakthrus were made towards socially-responsible public nudity, repressive forces went on full attack. One state tried to pass legislation which would have made nudity—even in one's own home, if children were present—punishable by up to ten years in prison. The same retail stores that sold movies depicting wanton death and mind-numbing brutality made photo lab customers feel like criminals if their rolls contained nudity, refusing to print copies, no matter how innocent or tasteful they were. Their commercially-released,

R-rated movies, with sexualized, often dehumanizing nudity on a nearby rack, okay; gentle, real-life photos affirming the sweetness of life, no way. Some called it the madness of the Beast that had much of the world in its grip. There was no making sense of it.

Dan Speers, president of Tri-State Metro Nudists, summed up the pity of it all: "For someone to tell me—especially the government authority—that I *have* to wear clothes, they're telling me that I have to be ashamed of myself. Government is mandating that people *shame* themselves."

*****

By 2005, the trend towards a viable freebody culture was kicking into higher gear. Proactive efforts to get more clothing-optional public beaches, lake and riverfronts set aside were succeeding. Free beaches pulled record numbers to enjoy the sun and surf, free of textile restraints. More men than women went nude, as had long been the case, altho numbers were beginning to even out as women empowered themselves and men eased off on idly objectifying them. Those who still clung to bits of textile increasingly wore thongs or G-strings, and men had their own brief variations.

Parts of the U.S., at least, were achieving the freebody awareness Europeans had cultivated decades earlier. Town residents took to indulging in the luxury of nude sunbathing on roofs, back decks and gardens more often—even front lawns, some no longer caring if others saw them unwrapped or not. The growing mantra was: "I'm nekkid. Big deal. Get over it." Pleasant weather inspired barely-there wear, token cover-ups for maximum body comfort and receptivity to the elements. Thong underwear had caught on a few years earlier, freeing the butt from double-wrapping, and now the next logical step emerged: In nicest weather people skipped underwear entirely—a thing few "self-respecting" persons would have done only years before.

Many veered away from needlessly constrictive, chafing clothes; simpler warm-weather designs forewent bothersome, dress-intensive zippers, buttons and buckles of traditional pants in favor of gentle elastic waistbands or draw-strings. Soft, loose-fitting flannel pajama bottoms and yoga pants were body-friendly fashion statements.

After winning much-ballyhooed court cases in several states in recent years, a steady trickle of women calmly, mindfully began going topfree *beyond* the beach and pool. Brilliant attorneys had successfully argued against the existing legal inequality which permitted men but not women to freely go in many public places without top cover. Now, in a dozen states at least, women could be topfree anywhere men could, so long as the intent wasn't overtly sexual. More women might have broken free of this dress restriction sooner but for inertia—if one is kept caged long enuf, one often stares awhile at a door suddenly opened before at last walking out. Also, men, besides blue-collar workers, seldom took advantage of their long-held top-optional freedoms beyond the water, except on hottest days, and if they didn't, women would tend not to either.

More women *did* take advantage of the new dress-equality law in those states by *driving* topfree, tho, especially in warm weather. Since the inside of a vehicle was more a private than public space—one's personal comfort zone while traveling—people were naturally inclined to get comfy. The fewer the clothes, the comfier, even with air conditioning.

As male naturists knew, if you drove topfree it was often an easy stretch with simple precautions to drive *bottomfree* as well without attracting any more notice, especially with high-speed, high-carriage, tinted-window travel on the open highway. One simply stayed calmly alert and kept a towel or clothing nearby to pull over the lap whenever high-vantage trucks, buses and RVs were close, and sat on an undone sarong for easy cover when wanted or needed. As I discovered myself one summer, there were few things that felt so liberating as hopping in your car buck-naked and going for a drive thru the countryside, hopping out, nude as ever, at your destination. Drivers had to remember to cover up on crossing certain state lines; reports of naked drivers in nude-intolerant regions still inspired high-speed keystone cops chases down the highway.

Whenever weather allowed, more of *both* genders favored wearing sarongs, those light wrap-around fringed cloths, done in bursts of colors and inspired patterns. Various men in some regions—not gay or cross-dressers—had at last rebelled against those prescribed two-legged cover-ups called pants, which, short of sitting down, required the ungracious, stooped over, one-legged dance to don and doff—and often crowded the genitals.

Males finally discovered the extravagant comfort of allowing their nether regions to breathe freely. Testes, needing a cooler temperature to be happy campers, are situated outside; jamming them up with tight, binding cloth defeated body engineering and definitely rendered the wearer testier. Maybe such a constrictive habit was a carryover from former times when men were always on battle-alert and needed their "family jewels" well-protected. Anyhow, many still seemed locked into that mindset, doing daily battle with the world; others were breaking free of it.

Long the exclusive domain of women, such apparel was branded ludicrous on Western man and brought about doubts of one's manhood. This, even tho similar wraps were universal in ancient Rome and Greece. Scotsmen with their skirt-like kilts were the exception. (Note of interest: a survey taken about 2002 at last revealed the naked truth on what was worn underneath: two out of three kilt-wearers wore nothing underneath. *Hoot, mon!*) By 2003, a Seattle company offered construction workers a canvas kilt—called the Utilikilt®—for holding tools and keeping jewels at ease while working. Kilts, sarongs and such allowed men's poor imprisoned genitals to breathe free at last. Someone came up with a daffy tongue-twister to reflect the sensitized awareness: *"Generally, genteel gentiles are towards their genitals genuinely gentle."*

All in all, the idea of a critical-mass acceptance of socially responsible public nudity no longer seemed *quite* so impossible.

Along with enlightened minds wanting world peace, an end to war, hunger, disease, racism, sexism, social injustice, hurting the earth and the animal kingdom…along with all these, people were increasingly okay with public nudity, thank you very much.

*****

A flash point was at hand.

And it was destined to happen in that fabled West coast bastion of enlightened attitudes and free lifestyles, San Francisco.

The City had already shone brightly twice in history as a beacon the world over—first the Gold Rush, then Haight-Ashbury. Good things often come in threes.

In retrospect, it came as no surprise it happened there. We know from basic metaphysical law the first collective energies of new inhabitants on new land forever stamp that land with their vibrations, its resonance to affect each succeeding generation. The first inhabitants of the City—and surrounding Bay Area—were local Indian tribes whose members often loved nothing better to do on nice days than roll in the mud and run around naked.

If *that* weren't enough: Francis of Assisi, the city's patron saint, after whom the city was named, upon rejecting all his wealthy father's worldly goods—including the clothes on his back—walked off stark naked in righteous dignity.

All in all, San Francisco had amazing potential for being the scene of lots of natives running around righteously naked.

And so, one fine day in 2006, in that fabulous, foggy town sitting on the edge of the world, freebody consciousness was about to make a quantum leap.

Ω CHAPTER FIVE Ω

Nice Day to be Naked

Bodyfreedom Day, Part 1

Not all the Greek runners in the original Olympics were totally naked. Some wore shoes.

—Mark Twain

The Bay to Breakers foot race had taken place in San Francisco every spring since 1912. It started to help lift peoples' spirits after the devastation of the 1906 earthquake and fire and also to draw attention for the town's upcoming 1915 Pan-Pacific Expo. Its predecessor, an annual New Year's race begun around the turn of the old century, went the length of Golden Gate Park. The new race course spanned the entire town, seven and a half miles, from the Bay near the Ferry Building to the breakers of the open Pacific—hence the name. For sheer numbers of participants, it grew to be the largest footrace in the world.

The 2006 race was extra-special, as it would help commemorate the Quake's one hundredth anniversary. Record numbers of participants and bystanders were expected.

In the mid-sixties, when I first ran it, it was a relatively straight-forward race. You likely wouldn't have made it 200 yards past the start line naked before being hauled off for indecent exposure. But times changed and the event increasingly became a city-wide block party, complete with mobile refreshment stands and live bands along the way—a madcap holiday celebrating spring, when the norm was suspended. To help suspend it even more, in the late seventies a daring registered nurse named Lesli Josephson became the first to run it in the nude; she ran it two more years clothesfree.

It's believed no one else had the audacity to run it again *au naturel* until 1986, when one Ed Van Sicklin did. Seven years later, in 1993, Sicklin formed a small nude-running contingent, organized as demonstrators, gaining strength in numbers—and an angle. Police randomly busted six of the group of seventeen at the finish line. Five of the six pleaded not guilty and hired an attorney, named, appropriately, William G. Stripp, who got their charges dismissed.

A legal fine point was established: It was their constitutionally-protected right to demonstrate in the nude, within exacting limitations. Besides, there was a public outcry—the town got a kick out of the naked participants, it seemed, or at least didn't mind—and the Frisky City's liberal sensibilities prevailed. From then on nude participants were *tenuously* tolerated by race sponsors and law as one of the more exotic participant flavors and generally championed by spectators. Bright-capped demonstrators banded together each year—demonstrating, among other things, how to get naked in public. They set guidelines for keeping within the letter of the law by staying on the route, not loitering, and keeping their act clean. Race sponsor *San Francisco Examiner* reflected the bemused acceptance in reporting one year that "...it was the naked people who prevailed: Naked nymphs, hula nudes, wizened nudes, nudes in every shade the sun could produce."

With the tenuous tolerance and public popularity, the number of nude participants climbed. At century's end, by which time bodyfreedom enthusiasts were joining in from all over, some 150 people opted to run or stroll nude. By 2005, over *300* participated.

*****

As luck would have it—or, in total synchronicity, others would say—a group of 900 naturists from across the country had come to town to hold an annual conference days before the race. Needless to say, they brought with them a generous dollop of body-positive energy. To cap their event—before joining in the run, as most planned to—they had won an okay to hold an informal clothesfree picnic and skinny-dip at one of the City's clothing-optional spots, Baker's Beach, by the Presidio. Some tried to stop it; it was one thing to allow small clumps of naked people there to sun their buns, but *900* at once... The mayor, who had been known to visit a free beach or two, defended it: "So they're naked. Bet most of you were born that way. Get over it."

The naturist group was a definite presence in town. Droves of vehicles were seen sporting bumper stickers and decals reading: **I'd Rather Be Nude**, **Loose your Clothes and Loose your Woes**, **Legalize Your Body**, **Feel Renewed in the Nude**, and **Nudists Have Nothing to Hide**. San Franciscans loved it.

Their formal convention proceeded, covering diverse topics like changing attitudes; exploring legal issues; sharing war stories and brainstorming stratagems for gaining wider acceptance. The group then had their much-publicized nude picnic at the beach, with plenty of volleyball and Frisbee tossing, inspired body painting and lots of skinny-dipping— the Florida contingent couldn't believe how cold the water was.

The *San Francisco Chronicle* gave the event straight-forward coverage—no smirks or mindless jokes—and included a distant shot of some of the group, subtly capturing their pronounced lack of clothes and apparent innocence of it all. Such positive publicity caught the public's imagination and helped create a surge of rethinking on the subject of public nudity. The article stressed the group's obvious comfort and non-judgmental acceptance of one another's bodies, no matter what shape.

Along with the predictably raunchy jokes on talk radio and the livid rage of those deeming public nudity an abomination, it appeared more enlightened minds were attracted to the idea, seriously questioning its fading taboo status. Why *couldn't* people be clothesfree more often? Why limit it to a few prescribed areas, free public lands and for-fee private ones, often inconveniently distant? The beach event had served to take public nudity out of the box long enuf it didn't go back in easily in the minds of many.

Most of the 800 convention naturists planning to join the run/stroll decided to adopt as their costume—no surprise here—the Emperor's New Clothes (altho one or two would rebel against what they saw as a predictable nudist conformity, going contrary and participating as mock "clothists").

Naturists were by then a diverse group—all ages, races, backgrounds, politics and lifestyles. While all were in favor of gaining more bodyfreedom rights, how much and how fast—if at all—to push the envelope of public acceptance was the subject of endless debate. Among the group was a more proactive core of a hundred or so. They sensed the time was ripe to give the envelope a decisive nudge; to that end they hatched a plan. After convincing the other 800 of its worth, they received tenuous endorsement.

*****

I was driving down to the City solo from my mountain home near the top of the California to visit old friends with whom I intended to do the race again, forty-one years later. Only this time I'd enjoy the surreal rush of leisurely strolling across town without a stitch on. Like them, my inner child rebelled against having to wear clothes unnecessarily. I had long practiced going naked around home, but seldom ventured out into public zones without regulation cover-up—not beyond safe havens of mineral springs and free beaches. I was a freebody novice, only beginning to resist the prevailing body-alienated energies from cramping my natural druthers to be naked more and not feeling weird about it. My interest stepped up a notch ever since getting an odd phone call from some publisher, wondering if I'd written a book on nudity. I'd said no but that I bet I could.

On the way down I made a special detour. If any place then open to the public on the West Coast had the jump on already being a brave nude world, it was Harbin Hot Springs.

Tucked in gentle wooded hills south of Clear Lake and north of Calistoga, Harbin was a nude paradise to some, a pleasant place for learning and healing workshops to others, an ultra-rarified cruising ground to yet others. A high-volume, 1,700 acre, seriously clothing-optional resort, it often attracted your more sybaritic Bay Area energies.

Its sometimes over-the-top sensual indulgence—one poolside sign, "No Sex in Pool," spoke volumes—was maybe only par for the course, at least for northern California—dubbed "the Future State"—given the state of American society. Too long we had hidden behind compulsory clothes which cut us off from ourselves and each other. Amazingly sensitive and receptive instruments that our bodies were, we were at long last able, in such places, to re-sensitize them and feast on the elements. In the process of intentionally coming together without clothes we enjoyed a good mineral soak and sunbath and reveled in the simple pleasure of being together clothesfree, frankly appreciating and accepting what we looked like beneath our mandated disguises. In essence, we were learning how to behave "normally" without clothes.

Getting any voyeuristic/exhibitionistic ya-yas out of one's system was sometimes part of the lesson. You saw enuf naked people and the forbidden-fruit, rapt fascination of objectifying each other's bodies began to subside (hopefully—some minds seemed permanently bent; at time I wondered about myself). It seemed there was often an invisible line between feeling sensuous and feeling sensual, as people once tended only to indulge the senses so richly and openly as a prelude to love-making.

I wanted a good warm-up dose of being publicly naked. There were other nice rural mineral spring resorts en route— Stewart, Wilbur, Orr—each with unique ambience, healing water and relaxed atmosphere; for an extra-strength, industrial-grade, *clothes-what-are-those?* public nudity experience, Harbin was *it*.

I found it humming with hundreds enjoying the day bare, hanging in and around the pools, sauna and creek-side camp sites—160 or more workers alone lived on the grounds, giving the place a sense of community and always working to tweak the already fine-tuned ambience to even greater heights thru imaginative landscaping and delightful little touches everywhere. That evening and many others I enjoyed soaking silently in the volcanically-heated outdoor Whisper Pool with dozens of others, making the de rigueur, silent gliding entrance down the submersed, railed stairway, the sound of the hillside creek magically trickling near by, the moon and stars shining thru the giant, overhanging fig tree leaves.

This was where, years earlier, I'd come out of the nudist closet, beyond the still-sunbathing, shy-skinnydipping stage, the same as untold thousands, no doubt. By week's end, being clothesfree felt so normal I balked at putting them on again at leaving, *the same as untold thousands, no doubt*—a woman there told me once she and her friends were miles down the road before remembering they'd better put their tops on.

Down in San Francisco, I landed at my friends' out in the Sunset. I was something of a novelty to them, having grown up with them there and then gone on to become a reclusive nature boy. They partly envied my tranquil lifestyle ("but what do you *do* there?"); I partly admired their wired energy and the town's rich cultural mix ("but you couldn't *pay* me to live here again"). Talk soon turned to the race. It was to be the first nude run for us all. I admitted I was turned on by the prospect of being naked in a high-density, clothed zone; it leant a sense of delicious daring. They agreed. To be naked and have it be okay amid tens of thousands of clothed people in a place where it could get you arrested any other day of the year was nothing short of mind-boggling.

No doubt part of my own excitement was symptomatic of some weird, convoluted mindset I was working thru, maybe overcompensating for being too emotionally wrapped by becoming more physically unwrapped. Maybe, walking paradox that I am, I was some sort of improbable closet exhibitionist then, needing to come out. I don't know. In any event, I was, along with most everyone else, trying to build body-positive feelings in a decidedly un-body-friendly world.

Adapting to the simple naturalness of social nudity—dissociating it from the hard-wired sexual link—probably involved reconfiguring more brain cells than the discovery the earth was round, not flat, centuries earlier; you *knew* it was round, but your whole life was built around thinking it flat. The deeply ingrained body-negative conditioning that taught us nakedness was bad could cling for dear life without something to jar it loose.

*****

May 14, 2006. Bodyfreedom Day

All that week the City had been in the grip of sweet, magical weather. Cherry trees ran riot with rich pink blossoms, acacia trees gave off their perfume and the earth was so fertile chamomile plants sprouted between sidewalk cracks. It was a warm, dreamy, sensuous, birds-are-singing-and-all's-right-with-the-world kind of feeling. One that made you glad to be alive—and begging to be enjoyed without clothes.

Come Sunday morning the air felt deliriously enchanted. Many runners only reluctantly donned their running suits after early morning showers. The deep-rooted taboo of being unclad in public was running into serious resistance in the minds of many who'd rather stay naked and luxuriate in that free, fine-tuned feeling. Why *not?*

My friends and I arrived at the bayside staging area at 7 a.m. We could feel the promise of the Mardi Gras-like spirit of celebratory zaniness—even with the chaotic milling of tens of thousands making busy preparations for the race. We paid our registration fee and got our number to wear, making us official participants and helping support a charity. Some of us were apprehensive about getting naked. For myself, I *knew* I wasn't in Harbin anymore.

"I can't believe we're actually going to do this! Are you sure it's okay? I mean, there's cops over there and—"

"Yeah, it's *okay*. Relax. I can't believe we didn't do it sooner. I mean, think about it. We've been like kids asking permission from authorities to be ourselves. 'Can I please not wear clothes today? It's so nice out.' 'No, you may *not*. Don't even think about it or I'll send you to your room.' Isn't that the way it's been?"

"Maybe. I donno. I *still* can't friggin' believe we're doing this!"

By pure chance, we found ourselves settled in next to the naturist-convention contingent, 700 strong and still dressed. Or maybe we were attracted by their relaxed, outgoing ambience, and had naturally gravitated near them. Decades of enthusiastically pursuing a clothing-optional lifestyle gave them a natural, grounded aura as they stood there, soon to be in their total element.

It turned out, I learned later, 300 bare demonstrators, distinctive by their bright caps, had arranged to join forces with the conventioneers, as most were naturists themselves and veterans of many previous nude runs; they figured the more the merrier.

You get 1,000 proactive nudists together on a day it's okay to be naked amid 80,000 or so clothed people—most only nominally—and interesting things could happen. Especially once the former decided they weren't waiting for the starting gun to loose their clothes. One moment they were fairly inconspicuous except for the occasional nude slogan on their t-shirts and tank tops and maybe wearing face paint; the next they stood out like so many bright, flesh-tone light towers amid a textiled ocean of humanity.

Maybe they disrobed early only to better catch the morning rays and get in the freebody zone, having little idea what chain of events they would set into play. Maybe they did it intentionally, wanting to be proactive beyond simply running/strolling nude, and thus give a boost to the efforts of their hundred activist compatriots poised along the route, knowing full-well the effect it was bound to have. Maybe a little of both. We heard both stories.

In any event, a bold move was struck. Nudity could be contagious. Whereas a naked person could feel self-conscious among clothed people, a clothed person could feel self-conscious among naked people—experiencing the same urge to conform. And the presence of the large contingent of veteran nudists, so relaxed in their skins, gave many sudden courage.

My friends and I now found it easier getting naked. Some of us were still a bit nervous, tho. After all, we weren't at the beach or by a mountain lake, or sweating in a sauna, but standing at the edge of a concrete jungle amid 80,000 packed, mostly-clothed people, preparing to run and stroll past tens, maybe hundreds of thousands of others, lining the route, all clothed; getting naked there felt incongruous as hell. We lost our clothes anyway—except our socks and running shoes, as our cities were *not* barefoot-friendly—and stashed them in day packs.

I was tall enuf to be able to see over heads and was pleasantly startled to see that *we seemed to be part of a straggled pattern of similar disrobing going on all around the group.*

Ω CHAPTER SIX Ω

Triple Euphoria

Bodyfreedom Day, Part 2

*Clothes therefore, must be the insignia of the superiority
of man over all other animals, for surely there could be
no other reason for wearing the hideous things.*
—from *Tarzan of the Apes*, by Edgar Rice Burroughs

As the nearby Ferry Building clock's minute hand inched toward the 8 o'clock start time, the sea of participants was psyched. Along with the usual serious, clothed runners determined to place were those who had possibly never even run for a bus. They were there to make the event a Mardi Gras procession with a West Coast twist by the elaborate, surreal and often comically absurd costumes they wore. Others have described them brilliantly; I won't try. Suffice it to say, people's fevered imaginations went into overdrive making them.

The unclad contingent was now about 1,200 strong and growing by the second. As best as I could gauge differences in body attitudes, some—mostly the commingled naturists and demonstrators—were standing proud and unashamed; some looked as if they felt a little naughty, and some naughty as all get-out. Myself, tho knowing it was time to make a stand for positive body acceptance, felt shivers down my spine and more than a little stage fright; what we were doing just seemed so *illegal,* such a mind-boggling departure from society's time-honored reality. I suspect there were quite a few that shared my general feeling.

In any event, we were all more or less determined to proceed and jog/stroll across town naked. We had the strength of experience and positive nude attitude at our core—dedicated naturists, many of whom felt so strongly about restoring people's right to *just say no to clothes* that they devoted good parts of their lives to the cause. We also had the strength of numbers: all ages, shapes, sizes, and degrees of fitness, all colors of the rainbow and every sexual persuasion, together validating we were indeed all naked under our clothes, just as we suspected.

My initial feeling of vulnerability, standing there starkers, began fading. There seemed to be a growing, all-inclusive acceptance for each other's naked state, warts and all. Considering the urban setting, people seemed pretty unconcerned about others' reactions to how they looked unwrapped—maybe because we were all in the same boat. It didn't seem to matter much whether you were an out of shape nude enthusiast or a *buff* buff buff. We were all who we were, humans in our essential physical identity. It was as if, once out of our costumes, we felt authenticated, validated as human beings, each unique, each with intrinsic value. With nothing left to hide outside, we felt it easier to be whoever we were inside.

Participants milling on the widening fringes of this growing clump of unclad humanity—vacillating whether or not to bare for the race—found themselves won over, doffing their clothes and stuffing them in their packs.

And so it had begun: Like a standing ovation, moving from the auditorium's front row to the back, a grand, inexorable ripple-effect was set into motion. Its ever-widening concentric circles of liberating vibration radiated outward.

In a matter of minutes our nude contingent had grown to 3,000 strong. Before the race started it *doubled* and then *doubled again*, and then *yet again*; the synergy created by this staggering mass of happy, earnest clothesfree humanity was staggering.

Carpe diem. We were seizing the day.

Anyone and everyone who ever had a fantasy of going naked in public; who was a closet nudist and wanted to come out, maybe seeking a fuller sense of their uniqueness; who was already a naturist and wanted to help stretch the envelope; who just wanted to shake loose of inhibitions or rebel a little—all peeled away their clothes en masse. Not everyone felt pulled to strip, of course. In fact, it was only a minority, maybe one in three. But one in three of *that* mass of humanity was still...*a mass of humanity.*

Unaccountably, people felt alright being publicly naked this rare day. It felt safe. It felt natural. A little *surreal*, to be sure. But there was magic in the air, a strength in numbers and an amazing, easy acceptance of each other. People felt daring. Exuberant. Deliciously *freed.*

*****

When the starting gun fired the air was charged with 100,000 megawatts of electricity. As we waited long minutes before the massive bottleneck of people in front of us could flow we consoled ourselves with the knowledge we were part of something quite extraordinary, possibly history-making. Others I talked to later said they felt the same thing; one told me she felt "divine spirit poured over us."

A sea of humanity, some 80,000 strong, were off—jogging, galloping, strolling or otherwise perambulating along Howard Street and out towards the blue Pacific. It was still a race for some, and they soon broke free, forming their own straggling running packs out ahead of the more leisurely crowd.

Among the surging mass of humanity starting to thread its

way across town were an astonishing 24,000 clothesfree people.

"I happened to be driving nearby when I looked over at a light and saw a solid mass of people, mostly-naked, surging by a block away," a witness wrote later. "I hadn't heard of the race and promptly lost all sense of reality the rest of the drive home. It was like something out *The Twilight Zone. Why were all these people naked?* I kept asking myself. At the same time, tho, it seemed almost natural in a way. Isn't that nuts? I was *all* turned around."

Most of our nude contingent went at an easy jog, each finding a stride, glad to be moving and getting the blood pumping—and wanting to get thru the often less-than-scenic commercial district quickly. This was a fun run, not a race, and most of us would switch to stroll-mode after about one-and-a-half miles, at the base of Hayes Street hill, and on thru the end. Some really got into sprinting, tho. A few of the nude ran barefoot as well, doubly amazing people: "Look, he's *barefoot!*" Lack of jock supporters for men was, of course, no problem, but it surprised many back then; unused to running naked, they didn't realize the scrotum automatically pulls the whole apparatus up tightly for safety and running comfort.

Another 10,000 or so of us were in various states of dishabille. Topfree, bottomfree, half-sarongs, thongs, tights, hula skirts, pajamas, baby-dolls—every conceivable kind of limited wardrobe.

In the rapid-change dynamics of celebrants' body attitudes there were dozens of reasons why some elected to keep a few clothes on. For many women, just going topfree was a stupendous breakthru in reclaiming personal bodyfreedom. For many men, it simply went too much against their grain to be fully naked in public, and in downtown San Francisco, no less. Too undignified—and perhaps fears of getting too excited being around one alluring woman too many.

For some people, it was practical concerns: Easily burned skin; needing body support; on their moon cycle; testing their comfort zones a bit at a time. Those in "sexy" outfits were usually either acting out fantasies ("I dreamed I walked across town in my Maidenform™ bra") or just being camp and showing how absurd some of the stuff really was. For yet others it was a matter of not wishing to offend others by obesity, anorexia, skin conditions, surgery scars, mastectomies, missing limbs, and such. And some, altho maybe already totally comfortable with their bodies, didn't want to seem to be conforming to the sudden avalanche of nudity and would wait until they felt their own spontaneous urge to uncover.

Others couldn't bring themselves to totally break the taboo. Despite the evidence all around them that it was okay that day, their internalized rag police wouldn't let them—at first, anyhow. One young woman, wearing only a thong bottom, when asked why she kept it on, said, as if the answer was obvious, "Why, I'd be *naked* without it!"

A large number, tho, who maybe *partly* felt like getting full-naked but didn't, were simply projecting self-criticism of perceived imperfections onto others: not big enuf, not slim enuf, not tight enuf, not built enuf—petty concerns perpetuated by a body-unfriendly society—when actually they fell well within the bell curve of your average human monkey. One might be a little plump, a little skinny, stretch marks, inertia taking its toll here and there, freckles, moles, hairiness…but your average human monkey.

While maybe only a handful ranked as "perfect" Greek gods and goddesses, many radiated an inner beauty that transformed their outer selves into something quite astonishing. People who the day before may have believed only the finest specimens of humanity had any business "showing" themselves naked were changing their tune. They had a revelation: A totally buff person in an ugly mood could be offensive; a person big as a balloon, in a jolly, self-accepting mood could brighten your day. As an old song went, "You're only as pretty as you feel inside."

A grand reality check was in progress.

We surged along happily, hanging a right up Ninth Street, crossing Market Street and hanging a gentle left onto Hayes Street and its dreaded half-mile hill. No sweat at a stroll; we geared down and kept on truckin'. Everyone, whether naked or in some abbreviated outfit, shared a sweet triple-euphoria: one part feel-good endorphins surging thru the bloodstream from running; one part pure delight in being bare-ass naked, or nearly so, on a nice sunny day; and one part rush of empowerment for flouting hide-bound notions of acceptable dress. All along the route people were subtracting clothes, adding clothes, trading clothes, giving away clothes, throwing away clothes—or staying bare—all according to whims of the moment, how heated we got hiking thru town, and the giddy realization we didn't *have* to wear clothes.

Many people among the twin rivers of spectators lining the route cheered at the sight of us and shouted support: "Yea, naked people!" Mischievous teens cooled us down at unexpected moments with their arsenal of Super Soakers™ spraying jets of water on us. People hooted. One participant remembered hearing a woman screech in amused disbelief, "Oh, my gawwwwd!" Some cheered and gave thumbs up. And some, as apparently happened every year, succumbed, loosing their clothes and joining us.

Actually, it seemed a *lot* of people were joining us, stripping and slipping into the growing river of bare humanity.

The staggered train of serious runners, far ahead of us, had long since loped up the long steep Hayes hill, jagged over to Fell Street, mostly clothed, a few nude like ancient, torch-bearing Olympians. After awhile, our huge amalgam of more leisurely paced—costumed, semi-nude and purely sun-clad—came into view along upper Fell Street near the Park's panhandle, astounding one and all for the sheer number of happily clothes-challenged.

Meanwhile, some of the naturist activists, rather than join in the run/stroll, were busy cueing up their plan. They had borrowed a page from Greenpeace. Having contacted proactive naturists by Internet beforehand, they found some with apartment flats along the route on upper Fell. As predicted, much of the media had chosen this area to set up. When the moment felt right—the crowds reeling from the surrealism of thousands of naked people cheerfully strolling along the street, parading around in the nude like it was their birthright —they unfurled giant banners across the houses' upper stories. **BEING NAKED IS NOT A CRIME** read one festively-colored twenty-foot banner; another read **BODY FREEDOM NOW**.

The largest, a giant twelve-by-forty footer strategically placed across the third story windows of a row Victorian where everyone, especially the media, was sure to see it, proclaimed:

IMAGINE A CLOTHING-OPTIONAL PLANET
Legalize the Human Body.

The rest of the proactive naturists had strategically placed themselves, lightly clothed, among the throng of bystanders lining the route where it wended thru the park on JFK Drive. Their plan, simple enuf, was to lightheartedly encourage spectators to join in. Once runners entered the eastern edge of the park, the City was largely left behind, as it was more or less pure park to the end of the course. Golden Gate Park was naturally the most relaxed and inviting portion of the route, especially with many of the roads closed to traffic, as they were that and every Sunday.

The park's easternmost area was especially an oasis amid the metropolis, being where the actual park creation began in the late 1800s; designers had pulled out all the stops. With its verdant grass, lush foliage, tranquil, winding paths and sun-reflected ponds, one easily imagined the area as habitat for faeries, earth spirits and water sprites. The area had no doubt often inspired urges on nice, sunny days to blissfully loose one's clothes, urges actually acted on during the hippie era with child-like innocence and forthright grace of people exercising divine right—*as if envisioning the advent of this day, forty years earlier.*

An unusually large number of spectators had chosen this stretch to view the festive proceedings. As the throng of mostly-nude participants surged by, the proactive naturists quickly lost their token coverings and joined in.

At first glance, many still seemed dressed, as underneath they wore elaborate body paint which imitated clothes. They were naked and clothed at the same time, wearing their bareness as a costume. Others had emblazoned across their fronts and backs colorful body paint messages in swirling lettering: **Dare to Bare! Legalize Humanity…Some days are just Too Nice for Clothes …Have a *Nicer* Day—Get Naked!** Yet others were walking works of art, having intricate patterns swirling over their bodies from head to foot.

As this sprinkling of pranksters trotted or strolled along, they beguiled spectators, offering friendly, non-threatening encouragements:

"Hey, it's *okay* to be naked today,"
"Come join us if you want!"
"It's your right as a free American, ya know?"
"Give yourselves something you can talk about the rest of your lives!"
One prankster, wearing only a freshly-made laurel on his head, periodically ran a little, stopped, and exhorted people in mock oration with out-thrust arm: "Good people, hear me! You have nothing to loose but your tan lines!"

"When he did that I finally *got* it," a woman said later. "They were like kids, playing in the sun, feeling zero shame over their nakedness. I thought, if these people were kooks, I want to be one, too, and got naked without another thought. My boyfriend was furious, but I didn't care."

Among those lining the route that day were, quite obviously, many who had already felt tempted to shuck what little they were wearing, but had treated the impulse mostly as impossible fantasy. As more and more nude people passed by many wrestled with last vestiges of obedience to the clothed-minded world and its programmed body-shame. With good-natured encouragements to actually go ahead at last, they did—nude in public for the first time since they were toddlers. It was, after all, a perfect day for an *au naturel* stroll thru the park; their birthday suits, too long in the closet, were in need of a *good* airing. Many undoubtedly experienced sudden shivers, feeling the sun's penetrating warmth envelop them, combined with a rush being free of clothes.

Between the delightful weather, the stupendous surge of unclad humanity all around them, the sudden bold banners and cheerful encouragements, people were gripped by an irresistible impulse—*and the ripple-effect continued outward.*

The lines of spectators began to resemble the race's intriguing mosaic of flesh tones and cloth dyes. Clothes came off like students late for gym class, like bargain-hounds cleaning off sale clothes racks, like slaves casting off their shackles. Some disrobed in slow deliberation, savoring the moment of deliverance as they tacitly gave themselves permission. Pronounced tan lines proclaimed how radical a departure from the norm it was for some.

Newcomers shared the expanses of grass along the route with those who had hoofed it all the way from the bay—who were now glad to shuck their footwear and luxuriate on feeling soft earth thru bare feet, their nudification complete.

In the more relaxed environment impromptu gatherings erupted everywhere, with music, singing and dancing. One group huddled and sang a spirited rendition of *Ding, Dong, the Witch is Dead*—the witch here no doubt being the Wicked Clothing Authority of the West; afterwards they skipped off, arm-in-arm, singing *We're Off to See the Wizard*. Spreckels Lake, right on the route, proved irresistible for skinnydipping and only the ducks seemed to mind. Its Portals of the Past—salvaged frontal columns from a stately mansion destroyed in the quake and fire—bore silent, sweet witness to the merriment.

As the contagious wave of released energy radiated out further it completely washed over the entire route's spectators, and any distinction between participants and bystanders fairly vanished. People thronged the park avenue in clothesfree jubilation, fitfully but surely migrating towards the ocean.

The only spectators left were straggles of stunned tourists, some disbelieving locals, stray pockets of foaming-at-the-mouth religious-righters, and, God love 'em, the Press.

"I Recommend it to Everyone!"

Bodyfreedom Day, Part 3

*I suppose we acquire most of our feelings
about our bodies too early, and in ways too complicated,
to make them easy to account for.*
—Charis Wilson

People, both bare and clothed, were only too glad to give their two cents' worth to the flock of media reporters on the scene. Among the soundbites:

"God, it feels *great!*"
"I don't understand it. Why are all these people naked?"
"I'm surprised it never happened sooner."
"I heard San Franciscans were different, but *this*…"
"We flew all the way from Austin to run it."
"It's like, way surreal, you know? But I could get used to it, like, way-y easily."
"If you ask me, these people should be *ashamed* of themselves."
"I can't believe how liberating it feels!"
"Just so much juvenile exhibitionism. People should grow up."
"It's a pure-D affirmation of being alive."
"Seems kind of silly to me. But quintessential San Francisco, at least, I suppose."
"Omigosh, It's *heavenly.* Why don't you join us and find out yourself?" The reporter, to the astonishment of her cameraperson, did just that, continuing her interviewing in the buff. She signed off with, "Naked and *loving* it, this is…"

For contrast, reporters caught the opinion of a hopping-mad

fundamentalist: "it's Sodom and Gomorrah! I tell you it's Sodom and Gomorrah all over again! God won't stand for it, mark my words!" This drew spirited rejoinders from nearby people: "God *loves* naked people!" "We're *all* naked in the sight of God!" He glared at them in righteous wrath as if expecting them to turn to pillars of salt any second.

The closing piece that would air that evening for KTVS, Channel 3, a cable feed for nationwide viewership, was an interview with a spirited young couple in matching sarongs. "When you think about it," the guy began, "I think we *should* have the right to be naked in weather like this if we want to. I mean, if it means not wearing this," he said, tugging on his sarong, "then—" but didn't finish, for he had unintentionally pulled his only covering off. He stood naked, looking sheepish a second, then grinned; as his girlfriend had promptly pulled hers off to match. In a burst of giddiness, they ran off hand-in-hand to join the procession, their brightly colored sarongs held aloft, fluttering in the gentle breeze like exotic bodyfreedom emblems, while in the background the banner proclaimed: IMAGINE A CLOTHING-OPTIONAL PLANET - Legalize the Human Body.

The network, deciding this was history-in-the-making, of a sort, broke with precedent and aired the clip that evening without pixelating their sudden lack of clothes. Capturing the infectious spontaneity of the day, the piece would show at least once or twice in much of the United States and overseas—before being mysteriously pulled. It and similar pieces were destined to galvanize the minds of millions.

*****

Meanwhile, back in Golden Gate Park: A tight knot of fundamentalist tourists, who had earlier raised eyebrows at various nude statuary disgracing the park grounds and made vows to complain to city hall, suddenly had living naked people *everywhere*. It wasn't a Hallmark Moment™. Other tourists were beside themselves as well—for running out of film. They knew the folks back home wouldn't believe them. And more than a few tourists joined in (when in Rome...)

People in neighborhoods bordering the park soon got word of things by phone. *("Jim, remember you said one of these years you were going to do the run naked? Well, you might want to come over here...")* A benefit carwash was in progress nearby; catching the drift and suddenly feeling overdressed in swim suits, workers continued on in the buff, in between turning the hoses on each other. People who happened by the route on foot or bicycles found themselves joining in; they walked off and peddled away naked, topfree or bottomfree, feeling sun-clad and more appropriately attired.

Police at first seemed to be facing a dilemma: It appeared the whole blinking town was going starkers. While participants had clearly skirted city ordinances by leaving the race route naked and "loitering," what should they do when tens of thousands were involved? Call up the Guard? Some wanted to. As it turned out, tho, spirits were so high and most people, apart from being naked, were so well-behaved, it wasn't an uncontainable situation. Police *would* end up arresting a hundred or so that day, but it was only those flagrantly disrespecting the rights of others and making rude spectacles of themselves, many of them drunk or wasted on drugs, who got hauled off.

The overwhelming majority of us were exuberant but socially mindful, all things considered. We carried on— purely delighted for the chance to experience such delicious freedom after a lifetime of cover up.

Like some impossibly-huge caterpillar, we pulsed towards the ocean.

Among the throng: A young couple pushing their baby stroller, a decal on the side reading, "Born Free—Born Naked"; an old couple supporting each other along (we overheard them talking: "Didja ever think we'd live to see the day, Harold?" "Never in all my born days."); flocks of women friends, saronged and topfree, chatting happily, looking as if they'd been transported to Tahiti without even leaving town.

There was the unofficial guest of honor: one of the last living survivors of the '06 Quake. A hundred-and-nine years young, his tribe of descendents flocked about his wheelchair, happily taking turns wheeling him along. Legend had it as a young man he was a member of the local Polar Bear Club, whose members braved the surf every New Year's Day. He often defied convention by running into the surf buck naked, much to the consternation of town officials. I spotted him briefly later, looking out at all the skinny-dippers in the surf with what appeared a quiet smile of vindication on his face.

We found ourselves singing, laughing and dancing along, the cooling ocean breeze becoming stronger. Tunes and rhythms were supplied by the many mobile street musicians sprinkled throughout: people played flutes, clarinets, saxes, harmonicas—there was even a nude tuba player who ompahpahed as he march-danced along. A troupe of drummers with strapped-on congas thumped out infectious rhythms that echoed across town. A mobile piano player aboard an ingenuous cart peddled and steered along while plunking out tunes, including a rollicking version of *San Francisco*. A college glee club, gleefully naked, reprised the song a cappella, with inspired four-part harmony; as they hit the last three chords of the bridge it sent shivers down my spine. They followed that singing *By the Sea, By the Sea* and then—shades of Woodstock—led us in spirited rounds of *Row, Row, Row your Boat*.

Our procession pulled towards the ocean as if by magnet, entranced, feeling indeed life was but a dream. My friends and I caught a powerful whiff of tangy salt air and instantly felt galvanized, running the rest of the way down hill, the ocean springing into view. Someone yelled, "last one in the water buys dinner!"—I think it was me; I was almost broke, so I really hoofed it. We felt the sweet sensation of air currents caressing our bodies as we sprinted. A giant old windmill, one of two long-retired alternate-energy workhorses once used for watering the park, loomed in the distance. We dashed across closed-off Ocean Highway and plowed thru the beach sands. "Wait, I *can't*," one of us joked in mock distress seconds before splashing into the Pacific, "I forgot my swim suit!"

Race officials, seeing the futility of trying to keep a handle on things, had abandoned the finish chutes, standing aside in wonderment. The spectacle of so much naked humanity pouring out along the long stretch of Ocean Beach was something they'd remember the rest of their lives.

There naturally followed the world's largest skinny-dipping party, altho there was no Guinness official present to verify. We were so pumped from running, strolling and dancing that the chill ocean water felt wonderful, its liquid magic steeling our newly-liberated bodies and causing tingles of inexplicable joy.

*****

A feature piece in next day's *Chronicle* read:

> They dreamed they walked across town in their birthday suits...but it was no dream...or was it? Yesterday a sea of Bay-to-Breakers participants and joiners-in blithely ran and strolled across town nude or

nearly so—turning centuries of the unspoken dictate "Thou Shalt Wear Clothes" flat on its ears.

It's become popular in recent years for a handful of participants to run naked, "demonstrating against the absurd U.S. phobia over the naked self." At some point yesterday the event transformed from a festive race-and-stroll into a cultural phenomenon of epic proportions. Never in recorded history has there been such an en masse breaking free of clothes.

Tho the mind-boggling import of the day hasn't sunk in yet for many, yesterday an estimated 150,000 people—together in the altogether—effectively transformed San Francisco into a truly Naked City.

Talk about The City That Knows How.

*****

And talk people did. Among the flood of letters to the editor printed the next day:

"It's an elusive feeling to describe, strolling across town *au naturel*. It's easily one of the most amazing, exhilarating experiences I've ever had. I heartily recommend it to everyone."

"What I want to know is: How come we only do this one day a year?"

"Until yesterday the very notion of going naked in public—in the bustling city no less—I would have deemed sheer lunacy. And yet there was some sweet intoxication in the air…as if the muses of old had poured forth from their grand amphorae a magical enchantment over people to open their hearts and minds into re-discovering (as I soon did) the simple, exquisite pleasure of enjoying the day free of clothes, and sharing that delight with others. I felt so liberated I joked to my friends I wasn't ever putting my clothes back on."

A college sweetheart I hadn't seen in ages was apparently there, for she—sharing my penchant for silly rhyme—penned and signed the following:

"We threaded along, among the throng, nude or in thong or bright sarong, singing a song, feeling no wrong (so sue me)."

And finally, this one, which began to capture the import of the day:

"…Together we made it feel it was not only okay to be clothes-free—it was *natural*, the way it should be. We each decided what clothes, if any, we wanted to wear… I felt we were part of history. As if we'd stormed the Bastille. That we'd dumped unwanted tea into Boston Harbor. We sure dumped our unwanted clothes, anyhow. Only in San Francisco."

*****

Of course, it wasn't only in San Francisco.

Amazing to relate, the Hundredth Monkey effect took place.

You remember the story (for a more apt analogy, I've substituted foods): Island monkeys at one time were struggling to figure out how to peel bananas growing there to enjoy the fruit inside without eating the peel as well. The more adept and determined began figuring it out and teaching others, then more and more, until, finally, the hundredth monkey figured it out and enjoyed eating the fruit, skin-free. At the very instant the hundredth one got it, the knowledge was *instantaneously* transmitted to all the monkeys on the island. Even more amazing, this knowledge then jumped *over* the sea.; monkeys on other islands suddenly knew how to peel bananas as well.

Similarly, we human monkeys had been wrestling to figure out how to peel away our *own* banana skins—clothes—and feast on the weather, without it being an issue.

Was it possible to remove our second skin without suffering discomfort by weird or obsessive reactions from others? Over the years many emboldened spirits tried. First one succeeded for a while, then another, then small groups, here and in other countries, determined not to be victimized by irrational, oppressive attitudes, making a peaceful, socially responsible stand for the right to go naked if they wanted.

That day in San Francisco the hundredth monkey—in this case, maybe the 100,000th human monkey—peeled away his or her outer skin. *Suddenly*, activating the spiritual circuit in the Over-Soul thru which everyone is inter-connected, the more attuned freebody enthusiasts *everywhere* psychically intuited the breakthru and peeled off their clothes the first chance they got. Lack of public acceptance had been the main thing holding many back and suddenly that dam was bursting.

As it turned out, much of the nation had been experiencing pleasant weather as well. Aware bodyfreedom enthusiasts in places as disparate as Tucumcari, New Mexico; Savannah, Georgia; and Kealakekua, Hawaii; felt the same spontaneous urge, out of the blue, in synchronicity with the people at the epicenter and instantly gave themselves permission to shuck their clothes wherever there was a modicum of friendly earth or splash of water—sometimes *wherever*.

Zak was so right saying it sounded like a hide-and-seek game that we'd been playing; it really was. In that game, there's the signal it's safe to come out and reveal yourself. In effect we had just shouted it in deafening chorus to the entire planet:

"Olli, olli, Oxen-free-eee!!"

Ω CHAPTER EIGHT Ω

Prometheus Unbound

Freebody Culture Takes Off

*I come from a country where you don't wear clothes
most of the year. Nudity is the most natural state.*
— Elle MacPherson, Australian model-actress

A body-liberation wave washed over North America—and
the rest of the planet—like a tsunami. Places that hadn't seen
as much as a streaker in decades, if ever, suddenly had
people unaccountably sunning, picnicking, playing in the
water, nude and topfree—peaceably, casually, delightedly,
as if it was the natural order of things. ("I donno, George.
They just all of a sudden quit wearing clothes. It's like the
town's gone nudist or something. Should we be concerned?
George? What are you doing, George? Don't you *dare* go
out that way! Oh, alright. Wait for me.")

The more part-time naturists and private nudists in other
locales received word of events later in utter wonderment,
and fitfully followed un-suit, each according to their own
state of freebody awareness and resolve. Finding strength in
numbers thru the astounding phenomenon unfolding, people
who formerly maybe only went naked outside under cover of
nite were soon taking their dog for a walk in the buff in
broad daylight. They progressed in due time from "Omigod,
I'm actually naked in public!" to "hey...*cool*. But *you* knew
that all along, didn't you, Gofer? Yeah, you did."

Many who weren't even closet nudists began experimenting,
going nude around the house. Expanding their comfort zone
gradually, they got bold enuf at some point to go outdoors
and sunbathe and garden, maybe dance and exercise nude.

Many surprised themselves in becoming committed nudists in record time. The pure extravagance of feeling was like savoring a ten-course feast after a long diet of bread and water. Some went so far as to say it was more fun than bad sex.

It felt too weird for others, tho, to try to break a lifetime habit and go about doing everyday things without clothes; society's internalized judgments and force of habit put up a fight, and sometimes won.

A curious thing: for the countless people who *did* adapt and embraced freebody awareness, *nudity* became habit-forming. *What became weird was putting their clothes back on.* People were out-and-out amazed and delighted how free they felt.

The sporadic nudifying of America and far reaches of the planet spread like wildfire before thunder-struck authorities could fathom what was happening. Those who seemed happily resigned to compulsory dress, thank you, may as well have been in some parallel universe for all their understanding of what was unfolding. Having forgotten they were human monkeys, the phenomenon by-passed them entirely. They were clueless, their inner nudist beyond reach.

Before long, significant numbers no longer bought into the thinking that wanting to be publicly/socially naked was aberrant, naughty or kinky. Realizing our freedom had been suppressed, we got naked with a vengeance. Some removed their clothes calmly, some exuberantly, some defiantly— tearing them off and burning them in ritual—but all with the newborn conviction we were well within our rights as human monkeys to enjoy our lives without imposed costumes if we so chose. We felt, with a mysterious certainty, that *the clothed-minded order was at long last unraveling.*

The transforming energy afoot was aided and abetted by both the more freedom-loving press and the more oppressive media—whose negative spins and dismissive downplaying ("...clearly a concerted effort by exhibitionistic malcontents to undermine the way of life of decent, hard-working Americans everywhere") were so sad one *almost* felt sorry for them.

The more liberal television networks instantly scrambled to boost their ratings in a new competitive war to integrate casual nudity into their shows—as had been accepted for years in Brazil, Germany, the United Kingdom, Japan and Australia. It was shown sporadically at first, as far right forces threatened sponsor boycotts if the networks didn't start kowtowing again to good, old-fashioned body shame. Soon, tho, the number of viewing consumers who *did* appreciate candid, tasteful nudity in programming, now and then at least, became so great that some TV execs told the self-appointed morality police where to get off.

*****

We wanted to believe we had finally and forever thrown off the yoke of textile tyranny that had enslaved us, that we had triumphantly established bodyfreedom rights for the oppressively wrapped masses everywhere, yearning to breathe free.

But nothing comes easy. Lamentably, the Bastille hadn't fallen.

The order of wise and benevolent body-phobic powers dedicated to legislating our lives had gone thru shock, denial, fury and resolve in quick succession. Regrouping, they knew they had to do something fast to scare the pants back on people. If not, their whole game might come undone.

The Powers that Were burned the midnight oil trying to figure some way to call on the Patriot Act, with its enhanced powers to regulate Americans' lives—some reasonably, given September 11, others unreasonably. If they couldn't dream up a case to link getting naked to a national security threat, then, by God, they'd go another route. They hastily cobbled together a federal anti-nudity policy; serendipitously, it was so rife with legal loopholes and had so little support from otherwise law-abiding citizens in some regions it would prove ineffective for a good while.

*****

Public nudity became like Prohibition of the 1920s: Altho drinking alcoholic beverages had became illegal, it didn't stop millions from blithely ignoring the fact and drinking in merry abandon, feeling a shared spirit of delicious conspiracy all the while. They concluded that making it illegal just because some couldn't handle their liquor was unfair to everyone else who could. Now it was the same for those choosing a far more casual public dress code; the fact some had such shame-drenched body attitudes they were offended seeing others naked shouldn't mean *every*one had to keep covered to spare them a phobic reaction.

Even as Feds had then focused on busting liquor manu-facturers, distributors and floating speak-easy establish-ments, they now focused on easiest targets: obvious exhibitionists; egregious voyeurs; and the more disruptive, in-yur-face activists, who wore their nude militancy as a uniform—and whose rage could turn off many, less-confrontational bodyfreedom proponents. Most people simply wanted the freedom to be themselves, not force anything on anybody. Even so, some admired their willingness to go to the mat pushing for universal freebody rights.

Chaos ruled supreme for awhile. Peoples' brain cells worked

overtime trying to reconfigure age-old attitudes towards nudity, working to dissociate the automatic linkage to sex. More than a few traffic accidents happened in the beginning, as people lost vehicle control on seeing nude and semi-nude people casually strolling down the street. Since this initially surreal sight was far more likely to occur in tolerant regions, where drivers themselves might be nude as well, it wasn't as bad as naysayers had predicted. Humans can be amazingly adaptable to changing conditions, even if it involved age-old, hardwired reaction patterns; it took longer, but the more aware adjusted fairly readily, no doubt due to the increasing vibration frequency of the planet, which, when not resisted, helped speed personal growth and foster deeper heart centeredness.

State and county policies were in flux, and enforcement varied greatly from region to region, despite the seemingly mighty federal stance. Some states, long down on nudity, readily complied with new policies, while others told the Feds where to get off. So, while in some places the nude who were discreet and accommodating to the rights and sensitivities of clothed people were almost invariably left alone, in more conservative regions even the most low-key, considerate naked could be treated roughshod—put thru the wringer and hung out to dry.

Until federal law could be effectively implemented authorities had a thorny legal problem. They had depended heavily on age-old common custom and shame-game to discourage people going uncovered, rather than having *specific* anti-nudity laws on the books. Now legions of legal guns unearthed every obscure law and ordinance they could find and bent current ones into legal pretzels in their efforts to stem the naked tide. "Public disturbance," "indecent exposure," "lewd conduct," and "obscenity" statutes were zealously invoked. To enforce them, of course, they had to ignore making *any* distinction between the new, mostly wholesome, nudity and the more common salacious behavior of a lower-consciousness, guilt-tripping past. Because prurient charges couldn't stick, droves of cases were quickly dismissed.

Even so, in the first year thousands, mostly caught up in notorious surprise government sweeps, were indeed arrested ("Loose your clothes, go to jail") and hauled off to the station on irrational charges (these, in contrast to naked people acting irresponsibly; a naked person drunk in public was arrested for drunk-in-public, not naked-in-public). But for every *hundred* arrested for the high crime of wanting to catch some rays unwrapped and feel a cooling breeze over their bodies, a *thousand* came forward to rally for their release—nude, of course. Jails couldn't hold them all. The offense was reduced to a fine. Clearly, something had to give.

Support came from a few elected officials, some of whom were nudists of one stripe or another themselves and resonated with the movement. They risked vote trades in Congress and even re-election for their pro-bodyfreedom stance; one actually walked into session naked one day to protest his colleagues' latest repressive bills, before being hooted into sudden oblivion. Tho they lacked the numbers to do much, they served to help legitimize the cause and reflect the credibility gap which emboldened multitudes of citizens to casually disregard anti-freebody ordinances. It was much like people used to blithely ignore posted speed limits, even tho they faced a high fine when caught. People then couldn't drive *fast* enuf, it seemed; now they couldn't get *naked* enuf.

Fitfully, in some crazy-quilt way, public nudity gained a de facto legitimacy—bolstered by those who were nude-friendly, electing to keep under wraps in public but defending the right of others *not* to, so long as their behavior remained socially responsible otherwise.

Millions of us pretty much "got away with it"—as long as we weren't in the wrong place at the wrong time, kept our wits about us for quick cover-up if need be, and observed commonsense bounds of the liberalized propriety. Unclad people in more free-thinking regions were almost guaranteed hassle-free nude recreation at beaches, rivers, lakes and public parks, both in town and country.

Of course, many larger towns, with their hectic environments, concrete surfaces, and often conservative politics, could be un-conducive to one's feeling comfortable in clothed, let alone naked. Perforce, in such regions most social nudity out-of-doors still occurred in the friendly arms of nature and on private property.

Similarly, many smaller towns, with its denizens generally subdued and set in their ways, were not conducive to letting it all hang out. My own nearby town was a case in point. It catered to the more genteel, well-clothed-and-proud, tourist trade, so authorities were quick to discourage any nudifying of Main Street. While skinny-dipping was a venerable institution for the many nature-loving locals and select visitors at nearby lakes and streams, it was only in the quieter, off-the-beaten-path neighborhoods that people went undisturbed when shucking their clothes in pleasant weather.

But in some larger cities with nice weather, good city-planning and open-minded traditions, nudity actually became fashionable. People got into going naked or in fanciful states of dishabille. Elaborate body paint became the new status symbol for some—painted by exclusive body artists—to replace showing off expensive clothes. (Would we never learn?) Those with money to burn and body shame to lose and wanting to keep up with the naked Jones's fast-tracked at intensive workshops guaranteeing "Prude-to-Nude in One Week—or a new outfit on us." Some, wanting to overcome their clothing obsession, attended support groups for recovering clothes addicts: "Hi, I'm Bob, and I'm a clothes addict." *"Hi, Bob."* Others, with bad diets and over-sedentary lifestyles, were inspired to clean up their act, upgrade their hygiene, and take pride in getting fit so they could join the fashionably nude.

Sometimes entire neighborhoods effectively became clothing-optional zones. One could rise, take a stroll, have breakfast at the corner café, splash in the park creek, sun a while, and later join a block party, all without wearing a stitch. Some carried light cover-ups in the unlikely event of a surprise sweep or if the sun became too intense or scarce. One learned to savor the freedom of answering the front door unclad, as there was a good chance the visitor was nude as well; if not, it didn't matter—unless it was your Aunt Gertrude from Omaha paying a surprise visit, or a door-to-door petitioner for the Clothes-for-Decency League.

Inevitably, people began waging friendly contests to see who could stay nakedest the longest. One long, hot summer a determined couple was close to breaking the record of two months, one week, when their luck ran out. Their minivan broke down on the road passing thru a backwater town boasting signs, "No Clothes, No Service."

A surprising number of people in colder climates took to being clothesfree more often. Unless the mind psyched itself out by resisting, one's body acclimated to the coldest clime. Birds of a feather in places like Boulder, Colorado; Bennington, Vermont; and Madison, Wisconsin, enjoyed nude skiing, hiking, and swimming together; even people in Alaska in their super-insulated homes luxuriated in being clothesfree. It seemed the colder the climate the more frequent sauna get-togethers; people ran out in 0°F weather, bodies steaming, and rolled naked in the snow or fast-plunged thru a hole cut in a frozen lake. Skeptics in warmer climates didn't believe such reports, but living an active outdoors life kept the circulation pumping, and finishing baths and showers with an ice-cold rinse kept the skin cells closed for much lower temperature tolerance. Some believed it was all in the mind anyhow—that we psyched ourselves into thinking it was too cold not to wear clothes, and so indeed it was.

The radiant sun's power to warm has always amazed me. In my own northwest region, which got relatively chilly in winter before the climate change, I learned a way to stretch clothesfree time by tacking up a reflective space blanket on the wall of my south-facing sundeck wall, angling the sides out on half-sheets of plywood. So long as a full sun was shining and there was no wind, it didn't matter if the thermometer read 29°F.; I could still bake like a potato and dispel the wintertime blues.

Scientific evidence of the health benefits of judicious amounts of sunshine was published in *Reader's Digest*, helping popularize and legitimize nude sunbathing. It was noted the sun's Far-infrared energy was absorbed two inches below the skin surface, there helping increase circulation and oxygen supply to damaged tissues. We realized then why sunshine felt so good; it actually penetrated *inside* you. The discovery came as no surprise to true believers, who always felt better for not having swimsuits between them and old Sol. Soon after that article, a variety of people who once thought nudism just plain weird began practicing it themselves wherever they could—back yard or city park— for health benefits. Many soon discovered a bonus: Being mindfully nude gave them an unexpected emotional and mental boost as well.

We inaugurated Bodyfreedom Day. Every May 14 for several years freebody enthusiasts observed the milestone happening with gatherings at beaches, parks and private lands. Fresh attention was focused on issues at hand—nude etiquette among the clothed and the extra importance of hygiene, for instance. It gave enthusiasts a chance to better muster social nudity in their lifestyle, being among kindred spirits, and offered some needed structure to integrate changing realities. The focus on all things freebody served to educate the masses; enthusiastic new converts were won over on the spot, and more than a few old resisters finally succumbed.

Booths offered the latest body-friendly wear and skin paints, body-liberation pamphlets, books, CDs and artwork. One booth specialized in signs, both printed and routed in wood. Offerings included: **Posted - Now Entering Freebody Zone**, and a tongue-in-cheek twin set: **We do not Discriminate against Naked People**, sold together with **We do not Discriminate against Dressed People**.

Another booth specialized in oversize t-shirts, window decals and bumper stickers. Some of the more whimsical messages:
* **Save Your A/C - Drive Naked!**
* **Clothes can be so Unbareable**
* **If God had meant us to be naked, we would have...oops**
* **Bare to Be Different**
* **We *Nude* You'd Join Us** (popular among veteran nudists)
* **I'd Rather Go Naked than...not**.

More serious slogans:
* **Emancipate Yourself from Textile Slavery**
* **Body Freedom is a Basic Human Right**
* **Government Has no Business Setting Dress Codes**
* **Wear Apparel at your own Peril**
* **Don't Arrest Me I was Born This Way**.

Enthusiasts held picnics, lectures, workshops, dances and concerts. Honors were presented to those actors, writers and directors who had done tasteful, natural, nonsexual nude scenes in their films and thus helped the public gain healthier body attitudes. A popular singer of the time who had long ago said, "I wish we were naked all the time..." happily performed every year. Other popular acts participated—one year a group known as the Barenaked Ladies finally lived up to their name.

One favorite comedian did an instant-classic routine in which he came on stage overdressed and affected supreme shock at seeing a naked audience before him. He gradually let himself be coaxed, thru lightning-fast banter with them, to shed his clothes. Coming full-circle towards the end, he spotted a confederate in clothes and launched into surreal diatribe over how he dared be so offensive as to wear clothes. The audience split their sides laughing.

In time annual observance of the day waned. World problems kept growing and nudity was rapidly becoming so integrated into the lives of those so inclined, it seemed less necessary drawing attention to it and risking renewed repression being too high-profile. Many of us, tho, remember those times fondly; we witnessed the changing social landscape and marveled at the positive changes the celebrations brought into people's lives.

Further Unraveling

Ups & Downs of Public Nudity

In nakedness I behold the majesty of the essential
instead of the trappings of pretension.
—Horatio Greenough

During that period of fast-shifting body attitudes people flocked to lakes, rivers, beaches, parks and mineral springs. There they could test the waters of social nudity for the first time, and the already-acclimated who lived in less tolerant regions could pursue their chosen lifestyle in peace. Nude-friendly public waterfronts installed open outdoor showers with multiple shower heads; people who at first felt on stage showering nude in open view of everyone ("Ohmigod, everyone's watching!") soon accepted them with barely a thought.

"Clothesfree," and "Clothing-Optional" became magical phrases in luring related business the same as "Fat-Free" and "Sugar-Free" had been in attracting dieting shoppers.

A steep learning curve existed for beginning social nudists, let alone closet nudists. It was one thing to sunbathe or sauna naked, remaining perfectly still and low-profile—Nudism 101—and quite another to move about freely around others, doing everyday things, unconcerned about parts of one's anatomy bouncing and bobbing, sagging or dragging. Leaving behind a lifetime of inert public nudity (at best) wasn't always easy and could actually be a little terrifying at first for those still loaded with body shame, even in freebody environs. Others, who accepted their bodies but still equated all nudity with sex, could suddenly feel they were starring in their own R-rated movie; in nude-intolerant regions it might feel *X*-rated.

One taste of how free and newly integrated it made you feel, tho, along with how much more open others were to you, and newcomers took to it like ducks to water. The exuberance felt allowing yourself to walk and run and work and play and dance in the buff without feeling unduly self-conscious was nothing short of miraculous; it was as dramatic a difference over mere sunbathing as, say, motion photography was over still-frame. In time, long-forgotten baby memories of total, unselfconscious innocence, of being naked and fully open to life, began to re-surface, and people *knew* it was a good thing.

*****

Many who initially resisted relaxed dress codes were won over for very different reasons:

- Sunscreen, body paint and temporary-tattoo makers were ecstatic as business went thru the roof.

- Less wash and dry cleaning to do, a boon for every family with a passel of kids, a big plus in times of time-crunches, water shortages and overloaded sewage-processing plants.

- Fewer clothes to buy, another boon for families—and everyone else. People were glad to stop helping finance new yachts for clothing corporation CEOs.

- As clothing production cut back, the glut of material and human resources once dedicated to supporting an over-clothed world were freed up for more vital use.

- Thrift shops and new-to-you stores did record business as they were flooded by clothes from those needing fewer, which were in turn sold to inveterate clothes-junkies ever wanting more.

- Energy needs plummeted in hot weather over earlier years as people discovered in foregoing clothes bodies self-regulated easier. They often felt fine with just a fan on. Easing the energy crunch helped avoid rolling blackouts from energy-guzzling air conditioning units.

- People who regularly skinny-dipped and cold-plunged in lakes, rivers, and oceans, or at least finished showers cold, kept comfortable with cooler temperature settings in colder weather, again helping save energy use.

- Changing consciousness towards the human body fostered healthier attitudes. The porn industry, pants on fire, was going down in flames; they could no longer exploit body alienation. Flashers were going the way of the dinosaur, and exhibitionists and voyeurs were endangered species. Sundry strippers in nude-friendly regions started looking for other lines of work, while more talented exotic dancers happily discovered they were still in demand once they lost any gratuitous bump-and-grind, as people grew to enjoy tasteful presentations of graceful nude dance.

- To the surprise of many, sex felt enhanced. Being naked for longer stretches enabled couples to gain an exquisite, fine-tuned sensitivity not possible otherwise, as it took awhile to loose the shadow effect of clothing muting one's sensual receptivity.

- Workers discovered if, on coming home after a hard day's work, rather than slip *into* something more comfortable they simply slipped *out*, the day's stresses melted away more easily.

- Rape incidents declined. As rape was sparked in part by a crazed obsession to reveal what was concealed, the drop was shown to be linked to the increased, more open body-acceptance. Other violent crime dropped as well, tho the links weren't as conclusive. For one, warm-weather domestic disturbances declined as couples and families felt more comfortable and relaxed out-of-clothes. Even some nonviolent crime went down—notably clothes shoplifting.

- Absenteeism declined as work places relaxing dress codes made working more pleasant—especially those that inaugurated Clothing-Optional Fridays. Business owners discovered not only did productivity increase but air-conditioning expenses plummeted in hot weather. At one mineral-springs bathhouse, in warm weather attendants might be bare as the bathers—except for employee caps—thus helping put new arrivals into instant freebody mind state, and making it easier for attendants to tend the blazing, in-sauna woodstove.

- Businesses showing solidarity with bodyfreedom enthusiasts garnered loyal support. A common sign in front windows of stores: "No Clothes, No Problem." Restaurants hoping to cater to everyone offered Clothing and Non-clothing zones, providing fresh sitting towels for the bare-bottomed. "Party of five? Clothing or Non-clothing?"

✳✳✳✳✳

Alas, the trend towards public nudity was met with resistance from every imaginable quarter as well. Some simply couldn't fathom it. Coming from the older school and perhaps not anti-nudity per se—maybe being comfortable naked in private—they couldn't feature people wanting to be *publicly* naked; it didn't compute. They thought it an unhealthy trend to be discouraged. And skeptics imagined every kind of scenario unfolding were such a dress option to become universal:

- The sight of unclad people would be bad for business— with notable exceptions, such as the nearly billion-dollar nude tour and recreation industry; nude ocean cruises for 3,000 booked fast. Running the material world required material-ed people. Our naked selves might be closer to images of our divine selves, but the business world— largely geared to material needs—had no use for such divine reminders unless it helped sell shampoo or skin cream.

- The business arena thrived on intensely competitive drive. Workers girded their loins, gritted their teeth and launched into the battle fray, dressed from head to foot in Power Clothes. A naked business person could loose that edge in a hurry. Even if some could conceivably keep their drive naked, others would be incapable of taking them seriously; clearly the wrong kind of naked ambition. Even businesses priding themselves on transparent operation thought opaque a good thing on this score. Businessmen daring to leave off, or even loosen, their constrictive ties to breathe a bit easier were seen as fudging the game rule's strict decorum; image was everything.

- Protests from one unlikely business sector—nudist resorts and associations—seemed bizarre at first. "Wild nudists are giving nudism a bad name," one lamented. Altho referring to young people engaging in over-amorous public behavior, some saw this attitude as businesses bewailing lost revenue when one could now go naked in lots of places—not unlike Nevada loosing business after other states legalized gambling. Similarly, when an association claimed "they are hurting the nudist cause," even tho people knew what they meant on one level, on another it was seen as a *conditional* support of bodyfreedom, almost as if wanting to keep nudism a niche lifestyle for people with bucks, on their grounds, hedonistic *or* conservative. Or otherwise keep their tightly-organized brand of social nudity dominant, rather than generically available to everyone, everywhere. Whatever the case, it was easy getting so insulated inside a nudist structure that one cried fowl when people went outside it. Such structures served as temporary, tho crucial, scaffolding, enabling the gradual, focused expansion of enlightened body attitudes, and many of us were duly shocked when the more self-serving ones dug in to try to keep the status quo.

• Relaxed dress codes didn't appeal to others because in that age of maddening conformity people often tried distinguishing themselves from the crowd by the clothes they wore. People loved to dress up, as we still do—some things don't change. It's as a Tunick photo-shoot volunteer said: "People *think* they're revealing themselves when they take their clothes off; they're not. They're revealing themselves when they put clothes *on*." We become artists, good, bad, or indifferent, by how we paint the canvas of our bodies, as it were, with clothes and accessories.

People enjoy choosing colors, materials, and styles to match mood, occasion, weather, desire to impress. While women getting ready to go out may still lament, "I don't have a *thing* to wear," in a clothing-optional world it's not the same dilemma. A counter-argument made was clothes blurred people together by camouflaging the unique physical characteristics which distinguished them from everyone else, that by trying to stand out thru their clothes they were in fact hiding themselves. There was always another side to every body issue, it seemed.

• Some felt it removed too much mystery. Keeping clothed for all but your lover kept the experience of shared nudity special and intimate. If everyone could always see everyone else's goodies, as it were, love-making would feel watered down. And, besides, partners' eyes might also get turned too easily; men in particular, it seemed, could be too easily aroused scarfing up the eye candy of seeing other women naked, and didn't want to tempt fate—or involuntary salutes—being around them. Nor did possessive partners, realizing this all too well.

- The time-honored game of conceal/reveal in luring and keeping mates would be rendered obsolete, they felt. Many had too much money and focus invested in wearing alluring lingerie for teasing preludes to want to give them up.

- Both sexes could feel less secure if their every body flaw—actual or self-perceived—was visible right from the get-go, before even saying "hi," let alone trying to win over a prospect with their charms. ("How can you charm the pants off someone if they aren't wearing any?" one wit wanted to know.) In a depth-challenged culture, one that fairly worshipped an impossible ideal of perfection, body coverings helped level the playing field.

- Far fewer women than men felt comfortable with it. Even in ancient Greek times, when male athletes participated nude, female athletes kept on a short tunic. It was socially ingrained in male-dominant society no self-respecting woman revealed herself to anyone but her partner, lest she loose her virtue. It came as a revelation to men lagging on the learning curve that many women who did appear nude or topfree in public, far from trying to lure a lover or indulge in self-gratifying exhibitionism, simply wanted to enjoy time without clothes.

- In a survey of the time, it was revealed some 98% of women felt somehow dissatisfied with their bodies. Either because they "let their figures go," or, more commonly, succumbed to the petty body-image angst of a body-alienated culture, many women weren't happy at the prospect of their naked selves being in open view, other considerations aside.

- A lesser but still significant number of men also felt uncomfortable nude. Some simply felt too vulnerable or awkward. Others had become as obsessive about their bodies as women, dissatisfied with anything less than hardbodies. If they didn't have anything worth showing off they'd better keep it covered.

- Those of both genders not sexually active who hadn't begun to undo the hardwired connection between nudity and sex might feel uneasy naked among those who were active.

- A shallow culture that objectified body parts and pursued "bigger is better" thinking could be as merciless critiquing a man's staff as a woman's breasts. For some it was too unnerving a thought having one's penis dangling there in full view for frank assessment by every smirking girl and size-comparing guy. Then there was George's Seinfeldian concern of "significant shrinkage!" after a cold dip (see Chapter 625, Episode 81 in Video Encyclopedia, 2049 edition). Anything with such shape-shifting unpredictability was perhaps best left under wraps.

The rising consciousness of *people's* liberation would lessen these concerns for both genders over time. Men worked thru socially-imposed gender-role issues and got in tune with their suppressed female side. Similarly, women tapped into their assertive warrior side, "taking back" their bodies and enjoying social/public nudity without random male lust crimping their comfort zone.

Other concerns:

- Toddlers, not yet socially conditioned, were natural-born nudists. They re-taught parents to feel relaxed in natural state, reminding the world how innocent and free nudity could be. Many parents, tho—even those who were maybe comfortable nude as family at home and even with friends and simpatico strangers away from home— remained too skeptical about the state of humanity to endorse any universal clothing option. They were duly concerned about the safety of their kids if allowed to run naked among the more sexually precocious of their peers—not to mention the pedophiles who still lurked.

Even more liberal parents set strict parameters on where, when and with whom their older kids could be clothesfree—if at all. Children entering teen years with sudden body changes weren't always keen on the idea anyway. Others who did take to it at times became closet nudists in their own homes; many parents either thought their kids' raging hormones better controlled kept under wraps and/or, feeling so body-alienated themselves, simply couldn't deal well seeing their kids naked—it could even spark incestuous thoughts. Others, on a more even keel, were concerned only about the flack uptight neighbors might throw at them—report them to the law, even—for letting their kids run around naked.

The U.S.'s penchant for periodic witch hunts over various perceived crises of varying actuality was deeply ingrained in the national psyche. It was then manifesting in at times off-target, ineffectual protection efforts against a very real child-abuse problem. Naturist parents teaching kids nudism in their own home were considered reprehensible by extreme right-wingers, as if the parents were turning them on to heroin, sinking to incest or "God knows what."

On the other hand, more body-positive parents, at least those living in more enlightened regions, allowed supervised nude pool parties, beach get-togethers and park picnics among friends.

*****

As the growing, socially-responsible public nudity diffused and transformed the worst of pent-up, unnatural fantasy-manias and body objectifications, the once super-twisted mind-state of society unwound—enuf to begin moving past its antiquated attitudes and physical self-loathing. People were still only human, tho. Casual appraisal and open admiration of one another's bodies was still there. But it was just that—casual and open—not the creepy, drooling, judgmental super-scrutiny that once put a crimp in anybody's efforts to catch a few rays naked. The two-sided coin of voyeurism-exhibitionism, corruptly minted in our minds by bodies hidden too long, was rolling towards oblivion.

While many people came to feel safe foregoing cloth when weather, whim and circumstance allowed, there was yet another basic reason others resisted—*sheer force of habit.*

Millennia of tending to keep our bodies securely wrapped under cloth made us feel it was the natural order of things—nudity, the unnatural. We were like institutionalized prisoners who were so used to being locked up they no longer wanted to live on the "outside." Similarly, we were so resigned to being "locked up" in our clothes living outside them held little attraction. Or, again, like the Borg on *Star Trek* who were one with their technology implants and grafts, we were so one with our clothing we felt incomplete without them.

Clothes were our adopted second skin, our constant friends, our security blanket in an unkind world, intimately bolstering, caressing, enveloping our bodies, providing private, safe, customized mini-climates. Our bodies became so used to such always-there companions we felt *too* naked,

naked. (The fact we equated bared backsides with a feeling of self-conscious discomfort is brought home by the word "embarrassed," used to describe that feeling.) People had become *addicted* to clothes, evidenced by the manic enthusiasm generated over the prospect of going shopping for a new fix.

Many people enjoyed immersing nude in water—if only in bathtubs—the sensation akin to liquid clothes for the pronounced, all-enveloping pressure it exerts on the body, even as it becomes all but hidden under the water's surface. But the self-same people had little or no interest in adapting to the subtler sensations of sun and air on the body. It involved re-adjusting a long-established physical-emotional equilibrium and experiencing initial discomfort—and an easier likelihood being seen by others and weirding everyone out—so why bother?

For whatever causes, clothes were habitual. People had become so wed to clothes it almost seemed at times they'd taken some peculiar secular vow to always wear a habit in public—shocked at the thought of being out of the habit. The Order of the Perpetually Clothed?

Still Wrapped Up In Ourselves
Last Days of the Old World

There comes moods when clothes of ours are not only too irksome to wear, but are themselves indecent. Perhaps indeed he or she to whom the free exhilarating extasy of nakedness in Nature has never been eligible (and how many thousands there are!) has not really known what purity is—nor what faith or art or health really is.
—Walt Whitman, *A Sun-bathed Nakedness*

By far, the biggest objection to making clothing optional revolved around a perceived sense of threatened decency. The fading social order saw its time-honored sense of propriety under direct assault. Since the only time its members got together naked in mixed genders was for sex, the turn of events was clearly a moral breakdown of society. In their book, what was happening was nothing less than a retreat into mindless, shameless, self-indulgence.

This perception was fueled in part by advocates of open sex. It was always a fine line how far couples could share displays of affection and/or lust in public before hearing cries of "get a room!" No question, it was easier getting carried away making out naked; without consideration of others' *reasonable* sensibilities, nude *could* be rude.

Then there were your rank-and-file perverts, having a field day, including the lunatic fringe of the movement—the so-called "nudaholics." These people acted out, nude, wherever clothed people were, mocking them, like monkeys in a zoo, with "whadayagotahide, huh?" taunts, and otherwise delighting in making clothed people uncomfortable.

Such nudaholics and the over-the-top public-sex proponents trying to legitimize their behavior under the guise of freedom of expression, caused grief to mutually-accommodating freebody advocates. Even tho it was a misguided minority confusing liberty with license, repressive media made tons of hay from every such incident, trying to paint the entire freebody movement with the same broad strokes: Buncha deviant exhibitionists; sex-crazed sensualists; no decent citizen, blah, blah... Media voices changed their spin as it became apparent many otherwise upright, taxpaying citizens were ardent naturists. Now they shed crocodile tears, saying that while it was truly regrettable a few spoiled it for the many, everyone had to suffer as a result, blah, blah...so keep your shirt on—and your pants too. And, hey, your shoes too, while you're at it...damn hippies. mumble, grumble...

On what was dubbed *the Nude-Lewd Scale* there were people at one end with outlooks so twisted they always equated public nudity with sex orgies. They either acted out as such themselves or projected it onto everybody out simply wanting to soak up some sunshine and socialize a bit without being wrapped in manufactured goods. At the other end were those with a holistic view of their earthly temples. They accepted the naked self as one's unique and beautiful human identity in the natural order of things, and, for the life of them, couldn't understand why people made a fuss over whether one was clothed or not.

Moving along between these extremes were greater and greater numbers, shaping a new bell-curve reflecting shifting consciousness. A 2008 survey in the United States revealed that, as in the earlier poll, 80% of people still had no objection to designated free beaches ("as long as they *keep* it there, for God's sake!"), but by then 40% were okay with socially-responsible nudity, and 20% *were* socially-responsible nudists.

People were throwing off trunk-loads of body-shame, false modesty and other obsessive, chronic body insecurities along with their clothes. Increased positive body acceptance—one's own and that of others—made social nudity pleasant, therapeutic and self-validating. People felt more human and alive. Shucking clothes bespeaking one's income, status and lifestyle allowed people to feel more honest, sensitive and accepting of one another as generic, "no brand" members of the human race.

It was group therapy on a massive scale. While it wasn't a panacea for the world's problems, it did help ease more than a few of them. People happier in their skins were more likely to feel positive and thus make honest, constructive contributions to society.

Opponents pointed out that, whereas in primitive places even "heathen" natives oftentimes wore loin cloths, we were so much worse for showing *no* modesty at all. To this charge it was pointed out that, if indeed humans had some innate modest tendency to publicly cover their genitals—and the point wasn't conceded—the tendency was eclipsed by being buried under too many clothes for too many years *not* to want to get totally free of them now and then. Only then could we begin to strike a new, natural comfort-zone balance.

Quick-response bodyfreedom activists worked at damage control. It was easy for those undergoing sensitive healings from feelings of shame and self-objectification to feel blown away by gnarly, stony-hearted nude-intolerance and some adopted militant attitudes in return, demonizing clothes and their wearers. Clothesfree proponents, knowing such polarization counter-productive, launched campaigns stressing everyone's right to wear as little or as much as they wanted without it being an issue. The slogan: **Wear it or Bare it - it's Every Body's Choice**.

The clothing industry was predictably up in arms, their unsold inventory build-ups an embarrassment of stitches. Their spoken argument: "It's throwing people out of work and slowing the economy." Their unspoken lament: "How the hell can we compete with *that?*" Indeed, many clothing concerns bit the dust—and good riddance, we said—as people quit wearing their too-often synthetic, constrictive, uninspired, overpriced, sweatshop offerings.

People opted for loose-fitting, natural-fiber, body-friendly clothes. They still liked clothes—maybe even more, since they were becoming *optional*—our friends, not our keepers. People wanted clothes that let them breathe and move freely and let the sun kiss their skin, that were easy-on, easy-off: wrap-around skirts, sarongs, saris, muumuus, pareus, lava-lava, kilts, tunics...and, for minimal cover-up, reinvented loin cloths—in a rainbow of colors, only $9.95, while supplies last. Savvy clothing concerns had responded with new lines to match changing tastes and thrived. Also popular: over-the-shoulder totes to hold light cover-ups and barest necessities for the newly pocket-less, and vending machines offering temporary, biodegradable cover-ups for sudden temperature, mood and event changes—sorry, no color choice.

$$*****$$

For years it seemed a never-ending battle between those thinking a legal, universal clothing-option was all but a *fait accompli* and those vowing adamantly, "not gonna happen. Threw 'em in prison sweatshops. *That'll* teach 'em." Two popular anti-freebody t-shirts: **No Nudes is Good Nudes** and

**I'll lose this shirt
when you give a word
that rhymes with 'naked'**

The realists among us knew, on sober reflection, there could never be any universal acceptance of bodyfreedom so long as man continued hurting each other and plundering the planet and perpetuating sorry environments. More sensitive people, at least, would remain uncomfortable nude except in natural, secluded settings or in private. As someone once anonymously said, "Love is when you feel safe being naked." Tho we'd made strides, much of humanity still felt too stressed to want to ditch the first line of defense between them and an unkind world. Since many city environments were so un-bodyfriendly, only the tenuous bits of nature in parks and waterfronts were attractive for shucking clothes anyway—except during roasting heat waves when body comfort might win out over propriety.

Even so, dedicated urban warriors kept taking it to the street, protesting for the right to be naked anywhere, anytime. First, people had fought for the right to be naked on their own private property, then at designated clothing-optional, public spots, and now, anywhere at all. "The best thing to do," one anonymous person wrote sardonically years earlier, sometime before 2004,

> would be to designate everywhere as clothing optional, and we could leave little fenced-in areas for the prudes to prance around in. Call them 'Prudist Camps.' They could peer out of their fences and indulge in their offensive "I'm offended" behavior whenever they saw a natural person walk by, without bothering the rest of us.

We reached a few new watersheds of tacit public acceptance:

Until lawmakers fixed the loopholes in their anti-nudity statutes, more tolerant states, believing federal government had no business trying to set dress codes, complied only with the *letter* of the law. Cops went thru the motions of responding to finger-wagging complaints. But if they determined nude but otherwise socially responsible people at least wore sunglasses or sandals—*anything*—they winked and told them to have a nice day; technically, they weren't naked.

A friend of mine was apparently out of luck one time, the peace officer reluctantly readying to cite her, when she suddenly remembered—she was wearing contacts. *"Have a nice day."* Similarly, you could drive nude as long as you "wore" your seatbelt. Then the loophole closed, states were threatened with cut federal funds if they didn't enforce the law rigorously and cops had to write up naked people found beyond the confines of beaches and pools whenever someone complained.

Various naturist-Christian churches budded. They believed the naked state had the potential to bring people closer to the divine state. Accepting the teachings of Jesus but dismissing as poppycock the notion of original sin, they held faith in humanity's inherent goodness when allowed to unfold in a free and nurturing environment, one free of negative, projected judgments attributed to God. They performed clothing-optional services and wedding ceremonies, held nude river baptisms, and set up intentional, clothing-optional communities. "We are made by God, and in the image of God, so how can we be ashamed of His handiwork?"

No far-reaching, iron-clad legal rights were ever gained, tho, to safeguard clothesfree rights on public lands beyond established free beaches and various municipal pools. True, people were freer to go about *semi*-naked than before— except in a few states we needn't mention—but being completely, simply nude remained too much a slap in the face of clothed-minded sensibilities.

Again, the more naïve optimists wanted to believe we were almost out of the woods, but those who diligently followed events, legislation and court cases knew that nude-lifestylers were a long way from receiving much equitable treatment under the law; the Spirit of Justice statue in the Department of Justice's Great Hall may have been half-naked, but she was half-*clothed*, too. High-profile arrests of some more-freewheeling nude celebrities were being made in efforts to scare people back into textile compliance.

A case was making its way to the Supreme Court to try to decide once and for all whether the Constitution covered being uncovered. Prospects looked bleak with the decision resting on nine people who appeared permanently wed to their long, black robes, but you never knew.

*****

The world seemed forever and a day away from ever achieving universal body liberation—or universal anything else—*when The Shift took place and changed everything.*

No surprise to us now. It took the cataclysmic forces of nature to change us—a planetary hot foot: The massive floods and earthquakes; the tidal waves, eruptions and windstorms and famine; and, ultimately, the earth's momentous shifting of its magnetic poles—all worked to shake humanity out of its mad ways at last and back into the arms of nature and semblance of logical, divine order.

As everyone knows, after the Shift we survivors were forced back to basic survival mode in our long struggle to salvage and rebuild civilization. Whether or not one was wearing clothes was the last thing on anyone's mind.

And so the universal acceptance of bodyfreedom became a footnote in history even as it was gained and we made peace with our biologic selves at last.

When work, weather or occasion demand clothes, we freely wear them; when weather, leisure or spontaneity allow being naked, we freely remove them. Clothes are truly our friends now, never our keepers—especially since we returned to fashioning home-made raiment more often.

The entire issue, in the grand scheme of things, seems irrelevant now, of course. Yet the fundamental right to be clothesfree was a *cause celebre* in the minds and hearts of countless people *so long as it was a right denied.*

In those last days veils, which had long kept hidden higher understandings on all levels, were rapidly lifting. Some veils manifested *literally as well,* as in the guise of compulsory dress, which we lifted as we came to understand and honor our physical selves. We could become impatient for the rest of the world to see the light, tho we knew it was purely a matter of time; that it came in our lifetime was a pleasant surprise.

While it was perhaps understandable that people, so long denied the right and freedom to be mindfully nude, went hog-wild at length, we can't help but see such overboard enthusiasm as all a bit comical now. It seems it was always the way thru history: The pendulum of social conditions swung from one extreme to the other in attempts to correct a long-term inequity. Thankfully, we have come to strike a natural balance on clothes-wearing.

We older folks treasure being free to let the morning sun warm our bones; it makes us glad we're alive. That peculiar time when people forbad one another from being naked has thankfully faded into a distant dream. Even so, I'll never forget the liberating joy of that day when the floodgates burst.

Sources

The lion's share of factual naturist information came from The Naturist Society's quarterly, *Nude & Natural: The Magazine of Naturist Living.* (Address: P.O. Box 132, Oshkosh, WI, 54903-0132. Phone: 920-426-5009. Back issues may be available. Memberships help support bodyfreedom efforts.)

Following are the *Nude & Natural* volumes and page numbers from which various source materials came:

* Bay-to-Breakers race: Vol. 19.1, p.99; Vol. 18.1, pp. 78-88; Vol. 20.1, pp. 66-72.
* "The Naked Guy," Andrew Martinez: Vol. 12.2, pp.21-24.
* Vincent Bethell and FTBYS: Vol. 20.4, pp.18-24.
* Terri Sue Webb: Vol. 21.3, pp. 24-28; Vol. 22.1, pp.5-6.
* Steve Gough, walking U.K. nude: Vol. 22.4, p.99.
* Sandy Snakenberg's nude S.F. skating: Vol. 21.3, pp. 22-23.
* Kurt Barthel and Richard Ungewitter, nudism pioneers: Vol. 12.4, p. 76.
* Burning Man Festival: Vol. 22.2, pp 25-27.
* Seattle's naked bikers in parade: Vol. 19.1, pp. 25-28; Vol. 23.1, pp.33-37; Vol. 23.1, pp. 33-37.
* S.F.'s Baker Beach: Vol 17.1, pp. 45-47.
* 1937 court case allowing advocating nudism: Vol. 20.1, p. 63.
* 2000 Roper Survey: Vol. 20.2, p. 4-5.
* History of The Naturist Society: Vol. 19.3, pp. 49-67.
* Quotes from Lee Baxandall: Vol. 9.1, pp. 22-23.
* Sex offender list for skinny-dipping: Vol. 19.1, pp. 20-1; Vol. 20.3, pp. 41-42.

Other Sources:

- Skinny-dipping as former norm: The *Nudist Idea*, by Cec Cinder, pp. 439-441, Ultraviolet Press, 1998.
- *205 Arguments and Observations In Support of Naturism*, booklet by The Naturist Society, Oshkosh, WI.
- *Therapy, Nudity & Joy: the Therapeutic Use of Nudity Through the Ages* by Aileen Goodson, PhD, Elysium Growth Press, 1991.
- Advent of the modern bra: *Uncle John's Supremely Satisfying Bathroom Reader* (number 14), p. 167, Bathroom Reader's Press, 2001 (don't be put off by subtle bathroom-humor theme; the book series is an absolute treasure trove of knowledge on popular culture).
- Advent of the miniskirt: *The Best of Uncle John's Bathroom Reader*, pp. 323-324, Bathroom Reader's Institute, 1995.
- *The Hundredth Monkey* by Ken Keyes, Jr. No copyright reserved.
- Real-life nude San Francisco run: Bare-to-Breakers® website: Baretobreakers.com.
- History of nudism in U.S: *Nudist Society* by William E. Hartman, Ph.D. 1970, Crown Publishers, Inc.

Bodyfreedom Websites

"http://naturistsociety.com" The Naturist Society. Worlds of info.

"http://bodyfreedom.org" Experience Nakedness Project; Body Freedom Collaborative. Colorful, fun site.

"http://clothesfree.com" International Nudist Association. (U.S. based) Brimming site. Most informal. Bulletin board forums non-members may read.

"http://spencertunick.com" photographer of huge public nude-groupings around the world. Some amazing photos.

"http://barewitness.org" scrapbook of living peace signs around the globe. Astounding photos.

"http://baretobreakers.com" informs and organizes runners/ strollers for San Francisco's real-life annual nude demonstration.

"http://fcn.ca/inf" I.N.F. International Nudist Federation. (Europe-based; choice of languages)

"http://aanr.com" American Association for nude recreation. Around since 1931. Formerly American Sunbathing Association.

About the Author and Book

Stuart R. Ward is an expatiate San Franciscan; the house he was raised in survived the 1906 Quake. Twenty-five years ago he moved to wooded, high desert land in upstate California, where he's since enjoyed a seasonal clothing-optional lifestyle. Living in a modest solar-powered home hand-built "without power tools," he's earned something approaching a livelihood wildcrafting sagebrush for purification smudges, gathering pumice stone, and working at a popular, semi-clothing-optional mineral springs. Long a wayward writer, this is his first book.

The idea for the central story event originated over 34 years ago, when he wrote a short-short story of San Francisco locals "feeling inspired to loose their clothes in celebration of the day and run ecstatically towards the ocean." The book was written mostly clothes-free (winter intervened twice), first by manual typewriter and later by laptop computer–generated 98% by sunshine.

$$*****$$

Extra copies of *Body Freedom Day* available from the publisher, **Infinity Publishing.com** by Internet, phone or mail. (information on copyright page), or can be ordered through **most bookstores.**

Copies also available **from author**: $12.00 each, post-paid, first three books, in United States and Canada, U.S. currency. **International:** $US18.00, post-paid. All orders check, cash or money order. (**Calif. residents** add 7.75% sales tax.) Please allow 4 to 6 weeks delivery time; 8 weeks overseas. For **faster air delivery** within U.S., add $2.00. International, inquire at post office.

(Volume discounts may be available for groups and nonprofit organizations. Inquire with author.)

Comments, suggestions, feedback welcomed.

Email: stuartsun@finestplanet.com

Author's mailing address:

Desert Sage Books
P.O. Box 389
Montague, CA
USA   96064

A generous portion of any book royalty profits
will be donated to select body-freedom organizations.